To Work Out or to Wed

A Sweet Romantic Comedy
Novella

Savannah Hendricks

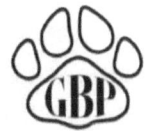

Grand Bayou Press

Library of Congress Control Number: 2020917404

To Work Out or to Wed was edited by freelance editor, Mary Dunbar

Front cover design by Cassidy Carter - author of *The Perfect Catch* & *Love on Location* from Hallmark Publishing

Contents

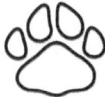

Chapter One

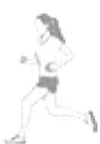

"We're a judgment-free zone." The gym's perfect-everything secretary smiles at me. Her eyelashes have more mascara on them than comes in one tube.

I locate her name tag pinned just below her sweeping bleached blonde curls. "Eloise, that's great, and I appreciate it, but I'd like to know my weight."

I try to keep my expression calm and polite.

"I think you look fabulous!" She smiles the fakest smile I've seen since Aunt Judy tried my homemade coconut vanilla cake. *Chunky, chewy, and smelled like old socks.*

"Thank you, Eloise. I appreciate your kind words. However, I don't see why you don't have a scale. I mean judgment or not, how do we meet our goals for weight loss?"

Eloise's pearly pink glossed lips pout. "Well, just by feeling great."

I sigh, and this time my eyes roll back. "Look, I have to lose at least twenty pounds in three months." *Okay, more like thirty.* I hold my hands out as though I'm measuring fat in distance. "Which may not seem like a lot, but it is to me. I need gratification, and a scale gives me that. Without a scale telling me where I'm at in my goal, how will I know if I'm even losing weight?"

"You don't have a scale at home?" Eloise picks at the glittery polish on her manicured nails.

"I do, but it's been broken for some time, and I haven't bought a new one. So, please help me understand how a gym doesn't have a freaking scale!"

Eloise points at the white plastic sign on her desk – JUDG-MENT FREE ZONE.

I grab the sign with both hands, snap the plastic in two, and gently set the pieces on the top of the desk. Wiping sweat from my hairline, I pivot as the rubber of my sneakers squeaks, and I storm out the front door.

After I slam the driver's side door of my cherry red Civic, I scream and squeeze the steering wheel. When Dane and I got engaged, getting married on Valentine's Day seemed like plenty of time, and now it seems far too soon. When I think about it, I couldn't be any more cliché if I tried: losing weight for my wedding and getting married on February 14th.

Of course, Dane has told me at least fifty times (*yes, I count*) that I don't need to lose weight. But I don't weigh the same as I did when we started dating. So when he adds, 'I love you just as you are,' he might as well be saying, 'I love you and your chubby knees.'

I glance down at my knees. Thankfully, they're covered by my way too loose black exercise pants. One day, I'll be able to wear the super-tight yoga pants like the perfect Eloise wears.

They looked terrific on the Target display rack, but once I wedged my lower body into them, everything possible puffed out from the top like an overflowing sausage casing. Not to mention the struggle I had getting the dang thing off. An employee had tapped on the dressing room door asking if I was okay since I kept bumping into the walls trying to keep my balance while peeling myself out of the yoga pants. *Think of the FRIENDS episode where Ross wears the leather pants—baby powder not included. And he didn't even have chubby knees.*

I give my knees a love pat and sigh. The sunshine is intense against the windshield as I start my car and flip on the air conditioning. Only in Phoenix can November feel like July inside a vehicle, even if it has tinted windows.

As I make my way home, I pass every fast food restaurant possible. Before becoming engaged and thus starting my wedding diet, I never noticed how many greasy drive-thrus there were on the way to my neighborhood. Now they stand out like a strip-club in the middle of nowhere. They might as well have a flashing neon sign: Bacon Strip Club—Nothing Goes Better With Our Buns!

There should be a petition for the number of burger places that can be on one street. It's clearly a conspiracy put in place by the gym owners. Feed them and make them work out. The cycle that keeps on giving to both businesses.

My stomach moans as though it's been without food for two days when I'm well aware it's only been two hours. I take a sip of my strawberry infused water because I heard it helps suppress one's appetite. *It doesn't.* Plus, my yoga mat came with the matching eco-friendly hot pink bottle, and it's too cute not to use.

I read if you're feeling hungry, it's usually because you're thirsty, and flavored water allegedly helps curb hunger pains. All it does for me is makes me realize I want to eat a strawberry cake, or a donut, or maybe a strawberry donut. It has, however, upped my bathroom trips, which means more walking back and forth. Clearly, multiple conspiracies are going on in my life.

At twenty-nine, I'm well aware of how many of my friends have already married, started a family, or at least are cohabitating, and as I pull into the driveway of my house, I'm reminded of this yet again.

My fiancé, Dane, and I don't live together. His parents are uber-religious, and we both respect them enough to not tick them off by moving in together before we're married—or that's the lie we tell ourselves and others. The fact is we can't decide who's keeping their house and who's selling. *It doesn't look good to others to admit this.* On the other hand, my parents passed away some time ago, so I have no idea if they'd care if we lived together before tying the knot or not.

I turn off my car and stare at the one-story house. It's not perfect. For starters, it doesn't have a garage. The paint is faded, and the roof may not make it another monsoon season, but it has charm and character. It's not a mass-produced, cookie-cutter home like most neighborhoods in the valley thanks to the sudden large spikes of people moving here. Dane has one of those homes, and I always feel uncomfortable in it, like he lives in a model home. And it's most definitely why we aren't living together—not because I don't want to.

For now, it's easier to blame his parents than our inability to address our different styles and tastes, although we're running out of time.

I climb from my Civic as Pear's barking echoes through the windows. Giving a quick wave to the neighbor across the street, I pull my mail from the mailbox. To passersby, my dog sounds ferocious, which works for me. Little do people know that he's nothing more than a hyper mutt who simply wants to cover them in doggie kisses.

"Hi, Pear." I set my purse, water bottle, and gym towel on the floor as I enter my living room.

Pear's tail wags at full speed as he spins around, banging into my knees. He drops the stuffed moose he brought me at my feet.

"I missed you too. The whole hour I was gone." I laugh because he has no concept of time. Pear reacts the same way when I come back inside from taking out the trash.

After I shower, Pear gets his evening round of fetch in the backyard. It's Saturday, so Dane is playing poker and endless games of pool at his friend's house. My best friend, Mallory, thinks it's odd that Dane and I don't spend all weekend together. I can't lie, I rather enjoy having a day where I don't have to worry about my looks or my fat rolls.

Living in Phoenix doesn't provide a lot of months to wear layers of fat-hiding clothing. It's hard to hide your figure in a tank top and cut-off shorts. *If you're thinking, well, don't wear cut-off shorts, we have to, or we die. It's hot. Open a 350-degree oven and stick your entire body in it hot.*

Mallory and I have been the best of friends since college, and while I value her opinion, she has a skewed view of life. Her husband, Jack, owns his own company in Mesa. He makes more money in one month than I've seen in my bank account in an entire year. Therefore, Mallory doesn't work; she volunteers. Mallory refers to it as working, but I remind her that unless she's taking home a paycheck, it's volunteering.

The other annoying thing about Mallory is she's perfect. Her Spanish-style colonial mansion is as sparkly clean as her weight is ideal. Jack's home every night for dinner and fully participates in every extracurricular activity with the boys. In fact, I've never seen them apart, other than for Mallory and my monthly coffee get-togethers. Jack and Mallory even have weekly family movie nights where Mallory makes homemade caramel corn, and they all lay on blankets she sewed. I'm lucky if I can remember to move my clothes out of the washing machine to the dryer before they start to get moldy.

I lean against my kitchen counter and ponder what to make for dinner. Pear laps up his water and flops to the floor with such drama he should have his own Telenovela. I run my hand over my neck, knowing full well I need to toss a salad together—or bake a chicken and steam rice—but the box of mac and cheese I've hidden in the back of the pantry calls to me, or more like sings like a jolly elf at Christmas. I hid it from myself because I figure I'd forget about it. I clearly haven't as I pull it out from behind the two bags of plain rice cakes.

"Everyone should have a cheat day, right, Pear?"

My dog looks my direction without lifting his head off the cold gray tile. I tear open the box as my cell phone startles me with the alert of a text. My hand jerks and I squeeze the box as a few noodles pop into the air like confetti. *Confetti cake, oh, with confetti frosting, yum!*

The message is from Dane.

"It's like he knows!" I shout at the screen.

Dane: How'd your workout go?

Me: It went fine. Nothing special. How's your day?

Dane: Mike beat me at pool. Twice.

I glance at Pear, who's crunching on the uncooked noodles that landed on the floor. The box of half-open mac and cheese is on the counter like a lighthouse guiding a boat to shore, and I'm the boat.

Whenever Dane has a run of bad luck, he always wants to hang out, and he wants to break from our Saturday apart tradition. I know it makes me look like a horrible fiancée, but I really want mac and cheese for dinner. If Dane comes over, I won't be able to eat any of the cheesy-noodle goodness.

Of course, Dane wouldn't blatantly say I shouldn't eat such a meal. Instead, he would suggest a different dinner. He doesn't have to say, "you should be having a salad"; I know he'd be thinking I should have a salad, and that is far worse than actually saying it. Sometimes thoughts are more potent than words.

Me: Sorry, babe. I guess you can't always win.

Dane: Of course I can always win ;) What are you doing?

I run my hand over the box as though it's a silky nightgown and squeeze the top of it in my palm. The noodles make soft noises as they rub together, and I swear Dane can hear them through the text message.

Me: Just thinking about dinner.

It's wrong to lie, but I haven't started cooking yet, so it's not really a lie. I could easily tape the box back up and make that stupid salad. My mouth is watering thinking of the warm cheese on my tongue.

Dane: I'm sure you're hungry after your workout. I'll let you go. Miss you and see you tomorrow night, Muffin.

Me: Miss you :-*

His nickname for me is because he loves muffins, and therefore loves me, but right now, all I can focus on is how I look like a muffin. And in my mind, that's undoubtedly the real reason he calls me muffin.

"I can't believe Dane didn't mention coming over," I tell Pear.

Sure, I'm okay with it, but my mind races thinking something must be wrong. Dane asking what I'm doing has always been a sign that he wants to hang out, so why doesn't he?

Taking the tape from the junk drawer, I wrap it over top of the mac and cheese box and return it to its hiding place.

"Great, now I want a muffin."

Pear watches as I remove the fixings for the salad—spinach, carrots, tomato, mushrooms, leftover rotisserie chicken, and a red onion. A surge of pride fills me as I put everything together. I'm making the right choice, even if I don't want to, even if I want the cheesy boxed goodness.

Once I have the salad mixed up in a bigger than average size bowl, I snatch the creamy salad dressing from the refrigerator. At least I can enjoy something with a smooth finish.

Making my way to the couch, Pear is on my heels and plops down next to me. He sniffs the air as I pour too much dressing over top of the veggies. All I can think about is the dang mac and cheese box as I munch on the spinach. It's firm and slightly sticky as the leaves fold onto my tongue. *It's like eating a damp envelope—not that I've eaten one, but they probably taste the same.*

With each bite, I contemplate opening a bottle of Pinot Noir, but somehow manage to finish the salad without doing it. After getting Pear a treat, I fold and pour myself a glass. *I waited long enough and I deserve a treat too.*

My stomach feels as empty as before I ate the salad. Cupping my wineglass, I squish myself into the pillows of the couch and fight off the thoughts of hunger.

The doorbell rings, and the wine in my glass sloshes as I jump from the startle. I make my way past Pear, who's switching between barking and growling at the door. Wine drops have stained three tiny spots on my long sleeve lilac shirt.

My heartbeat races as I look through the peephole. The doorbell has only rung a handful of times in the two years I've lived here, so I can only assume the worst.

"Maybe it's Dane surprising me."

I don't see anyone on the other side of the door when I look through the peephole. I bite my lip with hesitation. "Maybe it's something wedding related. Maybe it's a surprise from Dane."

I unlock the door and swing it open, my hopes high. Pear lunges for the security screen door, sniffing and barking.

"Quiet, no one's there," I tell him. "It's probably bored kids."

Just as I'm about to shut the door, I notice a small package resting on my welcome mat.

Unlocking the security door, I block Pear from escaping to either attack thin air or the package. The box is light as I lock everything back up and take it to the couch to open it. *Dane does like to surprise me with little gifts.*

Pear sniff-attacks the box like a drug dog on a mission. "Calm down. It's addressed to me." Even though I don't remember ordering anything. It's possible during my last PMS episode I drunk ordered something.

When I get past the packing tape and pop the lid open, I find two different kinds of gluten-free veggie chips. My face scrunches as though it's a box of dirty gym socks.

My cell phone buzzes, and I pick it up to see a text from Dane.

Dane: I figured you could use a reward for all your hard work at the gym these last few weeks. Enjoy!

I glance at the box and then back at my cell phone. "How thoughtful, he mail-ordered me a snack."

I respond with a "thanks" and a kissy-face emoji before tossing my phone into the mound of pillows.

Sure Dane is trying to be sweet, but he could've at least dropped them off himself. And who wants to snack on anything with the words FREE and VEGGIE on it, let alone both?

Pear noses the purple bag, and I pull it open. The scent of spinach and carrots wafts from it like a fart. My dog takes one sniff, backs up, and sneezes.

"Maybe they taste good." I remove a chip from the bag and take a bite.

"Nope," I say through the crunch.

My hand reaches for the wineglass, and I gulp half of it, trying to rid my mouth of the fart aftertaste. All I can think about is how well mac and cheese would take away the nastiness lingering on my tongue.

Chapter Two

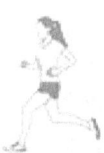

"Oh, this is *not* good," I whisper, stepping onto the curb leading to the judgment-free gym Monday evening after work.

A white grand opening banner blows in the wind. Below it is a bakery smack-dab next to the gym.

"Last week construction workers, today, evil conspiracy," I mutter to myself.

I lean toward the store's front window, spotting cakes, cupcakes, and cookies stacked up on the bakery shelves. Two tiny tables and a few chairs fill either side of the door that's wedged open. The scent of confections spills out like my fat rolls over the top of my workout pants. *Muffins.*

"You've got to be kidding me." I stomp a few feet to the gym door and wait for it to slide open.

"Good morning and happy workout," Eloise chimes from behind the desk. "Oh, it's you." Her smile fades.

"Sorry about the sign." I point to the spot where it used to sit.

Eloise glances at her cell phone, trapped in a glittery rainbow case. "The boss ordered a new one, and you've been charged on your monthly bill, Hailey." She doesn't even take her eyes off the phone.

"That's fair, thanks." I stagger over to the treadmill and take a deep breath.

The gym is about half-full, a mix of women and men in an array of sizes. While I know I'm not the most, um, ... voluptuous member, I'm also not the sleekest either.

I pick the middle treadmill in the row. Selecting which gym equipment to use is the same as picking a bathroom stall. It's important to always leave a stall between you and the other person whenever possible.

I step onto the treadmill, set the incline to zero, and punch the start button. My phone rests in the holder as I play a show from my streaming account and pop my earbuds into place. After a good twenty minutes, I'm zoned into a rhythm, but catch a man getting onto the treadmill to my left. I glance around and notice the man doesn't have the same understanding of spacing etiquette.

All the other treadmills are free, and this man has taken up residence on the one right next to me. But my focus travels to his lower body, and when I raise my vision, I notice he's gorgeous.

My hands grab for the bars on either side of the treadmill as my feet shuffle and slow down. I save myself from tripping and give an uncomfortable half-smile his way.

Hot Man on a Treadmill Far Too Close winks, and it takes all my focus to stay concentrated on walking, but I fail. My feet stumble, and I roll backward. Thankfully, I'm fully upright as I drop off the back of the treadmill with a thump onto the floor.

However, my cell phone, attached to the earbuds, has been yanked from the holder and is bouncing along the treadmill. *I should invest in Bluetooth earbuds.* The cord yanks loose from the phone, and my cell slams onto the tread, bounces, and flies toward me like a hockey puck. I pick it up off the floor near my feet.

The good news is I didn't face plant. Hot Man on a Treadmill Far Too Close reaches over and hits stop on my machine.

"Are you alright?" he asks.

I stick a hand on my hip and wave the other one in his direction. "Of course, that's how I get off these things when I'm finished. Don't you?"

He laughs and raises his eyebrow as though taken aback by my humor. We're even closer than before, and being aware of this makes me sweat more than when I was actually working out.

"I'm Edward." He holds his hand out. "Call me, Ed."

I shake it, praying my hand doesn't feel as sweaty to him as it feels to me. "Hailey."

"Nice to meet you, Hailey. I just moved here from California." He's still holding my hand, shaking it softly.

"Welcome. I hope you enjoy scorching summers." I pull my hand from his longer-than-standard-handshake timeframe.

Ed returns to the treadmill. "I guess I'll find out come July."

I let out a snort-laugh and instantly close my eyes in embarrassment. Ed is beaming a smile when I open them back up.

"What's so funny?" He punches some buttons on his machine.

"Summer arrives long before July." I snatch up my towel resting on the treadmill bar. "But, I guess it depends on what temperature you think summer starts at?"

Ed starts walking. "Ninety degrees." He shrugs his shoulders and hits another button, speeding up to a jog.

"Well, New to Arizona Ed, then summer will be here by March." I glance down and realize I've draped my towel over my left hand. My thumb moves to my ring finger. I can feel the diamond engagement ring as I roll it back and forth. I push the prongs into the pad of my thumb.

"Will I see you around here often?" Ed asks.

His ability to jog and turn to look at me without tripping or holding onto a bar is astonishing.

I'm blushing as every ounce of blood is now at the tip of my nose, cheeks, and ears. *I must look like I'm about to catch fire.* "You will."

He beams. "Have a great rest of your night."

"Thank you, you too."

I stroll past Eloise, still behind the desk, but this time not glued to her cell phone. She's staring past my shoulder, clearly impressed with watching Ed jog.

"He's so hot," she mouths.

"He's not bad," I lie. Of course, Ed is hot, but I'm engaged to Dane, who is just as hot.

As I climb into my car, I remind myself I'm lucky to have someone as good looking as Dane. It's not to say that I'm not attractive and that he's so-called marrying down or I'm marrying up. *The fact that I know those terms is immature.* I'm cute, like a cat kind of cute—a homeless cat who the entire neighborhood feeds. Sadly, I'm the only one feeding myself, unless you count the fart chips. Just thinking of them makes my tongue revolt and curl up.

I check the time on the dashboard as I turn the key. If I hurry, I can get home in time to shower and pretty myself up before Dane comes over—and hopefully, I can forget about Ed in that time too.

Chapter Three

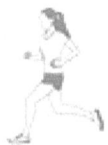

Tonight, I fold and give in to the box in the back of my pantry. Maybe it's because Dane texts me, canceling our dinner, saying he has to work late. I roll my eyes, we're falling behind on finalizing the rest of the wedding details and were supposed to have discussed some of them this evening. Perhaps it's the unsettling feeling in my stomach that something doesn't seem right between us. It could be because I feel guilty thinking about Ed way more than I should, or possibly, it's because I haven't lost any of the weight I need to, and it's already the second week of November. At this rate, I'll have to skip Thanksgiving. Good gravy. *Oh, gravy.*

The bowl of steaming mac and cheese rests on top of a couch pillow I use as a tray and binge watch three episodes of a reality show—shame on me, but I'm smiling between bites. I'm jealous of how confident the women on the show are, from dating to hanging out with their friends, and not all of them are the perfect Hollywood size.

I glance down at my body. I'm running a medium to large-ish size. Basically, I can fit into a medium, but then my "love padding" is on display, whereas if I wear a large, it's like a cheap version of Spanx. Can't see the "extra love" when the pants drown it out.

Pear snuggles up against me as it's chilly in the house. Burning all the extra calories makes me not only more hungry but warmer too. It rained today, so it's cold outside this evening. The two blankets that I usually have covering me, to keep from turning on the heat, are hanging over the back of the couch.

I pause the show and set my empty bowl of mac and cheese on the end table. My cheek rests on top of Pear's head, and he sighs with contempt.

"Oh, Pear."

When I lift my head, his eyes are closed, and he's snoring softly. I pick up my cell phone and send a text to Dane.

Me: I miss you. Hope work is going OK.

With each passing minute that Dane doesn't respond, my heart sinks. We haven't seen each other in two days. It doesn't seem like a big deal, we've gone this long before, but something just feels wrong. I scroll back through our text messages and notice there are fewer kissy-face emojis than usual. *Apparently, my second job in life is psycho-analyzing texts.*

Two years ago, Dane and I started dating. We'd both ended long term college relationships and had a lot in common when we met. Mallory had set us up through a friend, and our date nights were full of deep conversations at candlelit restaurants. We spent the winters visiting wineries around Tucson and the summers tubing down the Salt River. When Dane proposed at Cress on Oak Creek in Sedona, it was a fairytale come true. Everything we did was an adventure or romantic, until our jobs got in the way.

In our defense, our lives weren't overwhelming when we met, but now, they're insanely busy. With Dane working his way up the ladder as a marketing consultant and my job as a dental hygienist at one of the busiest dental practices in the valley, it's been time-consuming. It'll get better once we're married and living together—not our jobs, but less traveling back and forth to see each other will make life less stressful.

I snatch a wedding magazine off the coffee table and thumb through to the folded down pages. With my weight loss goal going oh-so-horribly, I need to wait until the last possible second to pick out and buy a wedding dress. Thanks to a limited budget, it makes this option more than reasonable. There wouldn't be any measurements taken, so a gown won't need altering. Mallory promised we would drive all over the state if we needed to to find the perfect-fitting dress in time.

Inside the magazine, I've wedged a check-list of wedding details. The invitations went out two months ago, but the flowers, cake, and music still need to be selected. Dane has already put his tuxedo on hold, and Mallory will be picking out her bridesmaid dress when we go shopping.

Thanks to a small guest list and Dane's parents' connection with his church, both the wedding and reception will be at a quaint, historic church just outside of downtown Phoenix.

Thinking about the wedding causes guilt to hit me when I glance over at my empty bowl. Maybe I need to go back to the gym tonight. I pick up my cell phone to check the time. It's already nine, and I realize Dane has yet to text me back. He must be busy with a client I remind myself.

"But it's rather late for clients," I say aloud and bite my lip. "I'm sure it's nothing."

Pear stretches his legs with a tremble, and then he curls back up. *Oh, to be a dog.*

I push play on the remote and try to focus on the next episode.

Unfortunately, a few minutes in, I discover the episode is about cheating. I pick up my cell and call Dane. With each passing ring, my heart races. I'm silently pleading for him to pick up, and when it goes to voicemail, I hang up.

"I'm overreacting. He's probably deep in an online search for more fart tasting veggie chips for me to eat."

Scrolling through my cell, I locate Mallory's number and hit send. She picks up after three rings.

"Hey!" Mallory screams into the phone. In the background, I can hear her three-year-old twin boys throwing a temper tantrum. "Hang on one second!"

The line's muffled as Mallory says something to the boys about Santa, and suddenly all is quiet. "Okay, sorry about that."

"Is everything alright over there?" I ask, the wedding magazine still open on my lap.

Mallory huffs. "Yes, now that I've threatened Santa won't be coming if they don't share their toys. What are you up to tonight? No Dane?"

I pet Pear and sigh. "I'm hoping you can tell me that I'm overacting."

"About?" I hear a wine bottle cork pop.

"Dane canceled on me tonight because he had to work late, but I've texted him and called, and he hasn't responded or answered his phone. And we still have to finalize some wedding details."

"Oh, no!" Mallory shrieks.

"Oh, no? What do you mean, 'oh, no?'" My hand is on my chest, and I catch the sparkle of my engagement ring. "What do you know?"

"Sorry, hon, no, I spilled some wine on my sleeve when I poured it. The bottle is an expensive one," Mallory says.

"How do you spill wine on a sleeve if you're pouring it?" I chuckle.

"Mom of twin's brain. It weakens all your abilities to function properly at the end of the day. Gosh, you don't think Dane is ..."

I glance at the picture on my end table of Dane and me at Page Springs Cellars last fall. "I don't know what to think, but of course, it's only bad thoughts."

"Dane would never cheat on you. He's a God-fearing man."

I squish my fingers deep into Pear's fur. "God-fearing men cheat too."

"Yes, anyone and everyone can, but not Dane. He loves you. And I don't think he would do that."

Guilt fills me, and sweat instantly forms. "Mal, I love Dane, but today ..." I pause ashamed of the thought. "I met this guy at the gym, Ed. He's gorgeous, and I threw my towel over my left hand."

"And?"

"And I covered up my engagement ring!" I lift my hand in the air.

Mallory giggles and then coughs. "You made me choke on my wine. Please tell me how this is an issue?"

"Because I ... I can't be suspicious of Dane if I'm suspicious of myself."

"Because you kissed Ed?"

"No!" I shriek.

Pear raises his head in protest of me waking him.

"Ed didn't follow the bathroom stall rule with the treadmills. He got too close and was so gorgeous I nearly fell flat on my face."

Again Mallory coughs. "I think I need to stop drinking wine while we're on the phone."

"Are you laughing at me?"

"Yes, of course, I am. The thought of anyone, even you, tripping and falling on a treadmill is funny. Come on, you know it is."

I press my lips together. "Okay, fine, it's a little funny." A smile twitches at the edges of my mouth.

"So, why are you feeling guilty about Trip-and-Fall-Ed?"

"I stumbled. Falling involves landing face-first." I sigh. "Because I'm engaged, and I enjoyed ogling Ed."

"Nothing wrong with ogling. Everyone checks out other people. And you'll be behind on wedding stuff right up until you say I do. Tell me what's going on with Dane. Is this something new? I mean, do you honestly think he's cheating?"

"I don't know." I slap my hand on the magazine, and Pear's eyes pop open. "Sorry, buddy." My hand pets his head, and he drifts back to sleep.

"Do you want me to have Jack find out what's up?" Mallory offers. Her husband is good friends with Dane.

"No, no ... okay, yes, maybe."

"Hailey, I'm sure you're overreacting, but I'll have Jack look into it so you can feel better."

"Thanks, Mal. Enjoy your wine."

"I intend to. Talk to you soon. And stop worrying."

When I hang up, an even worse thought pops into my mind. Maybe something terrible has happened to Dane. Perhaps he's stuck in an elevator or got in a car accident.

I call him two more times in a row, but he doesn't answer.

So much for relaxing the rest of the night, I take a swig of the wine I know I shouldn't have poured. However, what worries me more than the calories is how my thoughts are full of worrying about my pending married life.

Chapter Four

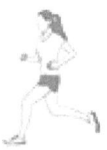

The last thing I want to see when I enter the gym is Ed. At the same time, it's also all I've been thinking about since I put on my workout clothes. The feeling is like sweet and sour candy, and I can taste the emotion of it on my tongue. *I know I'm wrong. I know I'm engaged.*

"Hailey, hi," Ed says from the treadmill. "You look beat."

I ignore my space etiquette rule and step onto the treadmill next to him. "I *am* beat."

"How come?" Ed showcases a perfectly warm and welcoming smile.

He's being a bit too friendly for someone I don't know. "Right now, I want to zone out and get my workout in." After the words leave my lips, I realize how rude they sound. "I'm sorry, Ed. It's just that work was horrible. I was up late last night, and I'm PMSing." My eyes nearly pop out of my sockets. Did I actually tell him that I'm on my dang period? *Yes, I did.* But when I glance over at him, he doesn't seem fazed at all.

"I have three sisters, say no more. If you're up for chatting after your workout, come find me. I'll be doing the weights for a bit." Ed winks and hops off the treadmill.

As I shove my earbuds into place, overly friendly or not, I'm impressed with how wonderful Ed seems. Dane always holds his hand up to me if I ever mention anything in the "women only" column. He didn't when we started dating, but he does now. A vision of me in labor pulses in my mind: Dane sitting in the waiting room while I'm delivering the baby, alone.

I turn my focus to the show on my phone as my walk turns into a jog. I need to step up my workouts, push myself further and harder. Weddings are about sacrifices. *Wait that doesn't sound right.* Marriages are about sacrifices; weddings are about being pretty. *That still sounds wrong.*

Sweat pours from me like a faucet and my breath labors. By the time I step off the treadmill, I'm not sure the tiny towel I brought will be enough.

"Great workout," Ed cheers from behind me. "You were zoned in."

"I needed it." After wiping the sweat off my face, I think about how awful I must look at the moment. My make-up is gone. My face is flushed. *I'm basically a hot-from-the-oven muffin.*

"Do you wanna grab something to eat next door?" Ed asks with a black towel draped over his muscular shoulders.

I'm so delirious from my intense workout and worrying about how I look that I don't realize I've agreed until Ed and I are seated at the bakery next door. The scent of chocolate and vanilla engulfs me like a wine buzz.

"Thanks," I say to Ed as he hands me an ice-cold bottle of water. The plastic crinkles as I suck half of it down in a long gulp.

A lady in an emerald apron comes around the corner. She's carrying a jumbo chocolate cupcake on a plate and sets it between Ed and me on the table.

"Enjoy," she chimes before walking away.

My eyes grow wide at the treat in front of us. I try to remember who ordered it, or if I was a helpless bystander.

Ed takes a fork and uses it to cut the cupcake precisely in half (*my measurement radar with sweets is superbly accurate*) and separates it. He hands me a fork, and I don't hesitate—but I should.

"I really can't eat this." I squeeze my fork. "It defeats the whole point of working out."

"You can."

"Yes, I can, and I want to but, no, I shouldn't."

"Moderation is the key to a happy life." Ed shoves a bite into his mouth.

"Do you mean to tell me you got *that* body from eating in moderation?" I ask, using my fork to point at him.

I give in because having a cupcake inches from me is too hard to resist. *If I can't resist a hidden box of mac and cheese, there was never any hope for this cupcake.*

I fork a piece and slide the chocolatey bite into my mouth. The creamy frosting glides across my lips, and I fight an urge to moan in delight. The cake crumbles and mixes with the sweetness of the frosting as I swallow. *Oh my goodness, that was yummy.*

Ed looks down at his body. "I didn't always look like this. I was quite a chunker."

I choke on a bit of cupcake and clear my throat. "You, chunky?"

He nods. "Yes. I wasn't obese, but I wasn't healthy. I made a lifestyle change so I could enjoy my life as well as hopefully live longer."

"Well, I'm just trying to fit into a decent size wedding dress."

"Shouldn't you be focused on your wedding? And less about your vanity?" Ed looks in the direction of my engagement ring. And without missing a beat, he asks, "When's the big date?"

"Valentine's Day." *My vanity? Gosh, am I that person?* "I'm not trying to sound vain. I must look appropriate. It's a wedding, my wedding. A once in a lifetime event." *Hopefully.* "Weddings are about vanity."

Okay, I'm arrogant, and that comment was worthy of an eye roll.

"Lucky man." Ed shoves another bite of chocolatey goodness into his mouth, and I watch him as though I don't have the other half in front of me. "So, that's why you look beat?"

I sigh and sit back; the fork rests in my hand. "It took my fiancé all of five hours to return my calls last night. I spent the entire time worried he'd died in an elevator or was cheating on me."

"And he didn't die, but was he?" Ed points the fork at me.

"That's the problem." I lean forward and nibble my lip.

Chapter Five

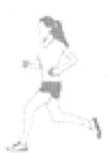

"**A**re we going to need a second cupcake?" Ed asks and holds his fork up like a sword.

"No," I say, unconvincingly.

"Was he cheating?"

My fork pokes at the minuscule crumbs leftover from my half of the chocolatey goodness. "I never thought of myself as a needy girl, but when I called my fiancé and he didn't answer, and he didn't text me back ... " I twist the fork between my fingers and lean forward. "I'm that girl."

Ed crosses his arms over his chest and leans back in the chair. "I don't think wanting a magnanimous relationship is a bad thing. And you found out that his meeting ran longer than expected?"

"When he finally got back to me, he claimed he'd put his cell phone on silent. That he needed to focus on work."

"What if there was an emergency and you needed to get a hold of him?" Ed suggests.

I throw my hands up in the air. "Exactly."

"When you grow up with sisters, you learn a thing or two about how men and women are different." Ed rests his elbows on the table. "And therefore, how each of us has to tweak some habits to keep the other from losing their mind."

His biceps showcase themselves like angels from heaven, and I glance at my ring to remind myself I can't be ogling Ed, especially while I'm complaining about Dane's possible infidelity.

I give my head a slight shake as if to get rid of the thought. "Tell me about Ed, what do you do for a living?"

He leans back in the chair. "I'm a high school teacher, chemistry."

"Stressful?"

"Depends ... sometimes." Ed itches his right tricep. "I have a great group of students right now, but I can't say the same for last year."

"So, all is well now with Dane?" He takes a sip of water.

My thumb twists my ring around my finger, playing with it. "I guess. My best friend, Mallory, her husband is friends with Dane and is going to do some digging around. Of course, putting his phone on silent doesn't seem like much of an excuse for me to think something is going on. It's just ..."

"You're concerned. And it's forcing your thoughts to link into how behind you are on the wedding details."

Ed hit the nail right on the head, and my shoulders slump.

I frown. "We, that is to say, Dane and I, seem to be slipping away from each other over the last few months." I spot two fabulous wedding cakes in the display case to the left of Ed. "My fiancé is good looking, and I'm," I flick my hand in my direction, "this."

I expect Ed to say something flattering, but instead, he stares at me. "And you don't think you're worthy of him?"

"Dane says he loves me just as I am, but how can that be possible? I'm fat."

Again, I expect Ed to disagree, to tell me I'm wrong. I need him to disagree. I want him to say to me that I'm not fat, but he just keeps staring.

Finally, he says, "And losing weight would make you happy, and you'd feel better? Like if he's cheating, then it's not because of how you look."

Words start to form, but I pause, holding them back. Ed's right, and I can tell he must be an amazing brother to his sisters. He's honed his women-conversation skills to a Hallmark level. Every man I've ever known has jumped in with a quick, "You're pretty, don't worry." Instead, Ed's not passing judgment toward Dane or me. The truth is, I want him to make me feel better and tell me he finds me attractive, but, gosh, I hate myself for thinking any of it.

"I guess so; I mean, who doesn't want a beautiful woman?" I ask, still craving Ed's response.

"Don't become vain through assumptions. Beauty is different to everyone. Dane wouldn't be marrying you if he didn't find you beautiful."

"But it doesn't mean he wouldn't cheat, and it doesn't explain why we can't decide on anything that has to do with getting married."

"I suppose, yet it doesn't mean you won't either." Ed screws the lid on his water bottle. "Have you thought about asking Dane what's going on? Put everything on the table?"

His words cause me to lose my breath because he's suggesting something I don't want to do. What if, in doing that, we figure out we shouldn't be together? I focus on my breathing without making it look obvious.

"As in, ask him flat-out if he's cheating on me?" I cross my arms and huff.

"Why not? If you're marrying him in a few months, you should be able to talk to him about anything. Confront him about why you're undecided on your wedding choices."

My lips form a pout as I ponder what Ed said. "Yes, you're right about that, but it doesn't make it easy to do."

"Of course not. But it's better to know than to look like you've been without sleep for days. Carrying the extra weight of the unknown will damage your heart more than any juicy steak will."

Oh, steak.

I run my hand through my low ponytail. "Do I look that bad?"

"I don't think you could ever look bad, but you do look tired." Ed half-heartedly smiles.

His words stand out in all my messed up thoughts. Knowing that someone, not engaged to me, thinks I'm at least not too terribly ugly gives me hope. Maybe I overreacted about Dane's disappearance last night after all.

"Thanks for the chat, and the cupcake. I do appreciate it." I stand up from my chair.

Ed stands too, and a part of me doesn't want to leave. There's something special about being around him—the comfort of being able to be me, all the good and the bad.

"It's been my pleasure. Get a good night's sleep." Ed holds the bakery shop door open for me as we exit. "I plan to outrun you on the treadmill tomorrow."

I laugh and toss the keys in my hand. "Oh, really? What makes you think I'm capable of beating you at anything?"

"You're a lot stronger than you give yourself credit for, Hailey."

Chapter Six

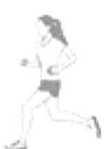

I squeeze my hands into fists until they hurt, and then I let go. Ed's words linger in my memory as I sit next to Dane on the couch an hour later, but I don't know if I'm angry with myself or the unknown. I've been fighting off tears of frustration with my weight.

"I had such an amazing hike this morning, these few pounds I somehow gained will be gone in a flash." Dane jabs his fork into his green beans. "Did you have a good workout?"

Tonight's dinner consists of sauce-less grilled chicken and green beans. Otherwise known as Boring Dinner 101. *And I thought I already graduated from college.* Visions of how great mashed potatoes, barbeque sauce, and a buttered roll would go with it dance in my thoughts. At least I have the simple pleasure of a small glass of Cab to enjoy. *Five teeny-tiny ounces.*

"Yes, it was good." Of course, I can't mention the half of a cupcake I shared with Ed, let alone that I spent time with another man. Not that I'd done anything wrong. Talking and having a snack is nothing forbidden, but the fact that I find Ed attractive seems like I should never have allowed myself to spend any time with him, cupcake or not. Telling either to Dane seems like a bad idea.

"That's great. I'm glad to hear you're still moving forward with your goal. It's not easy with our work schedules. I know I'm beat at the end of the day." Dane takes a sip of his Cab and stares at the television.

We're watching some type of sci-fi action show that's Dane's favorite. No matter how hard I try, I can't get into the storyline and find myself critiquing their makeup and costumes instead of following along.

"We need to nail down the flowers, music, and cake." I munch on a green bean. "There is a new bakery that opened up next to my gym, and they had some impressive ones on display."

"You went to look around?" His voice is taut.

I swallow and clear my throat. "I'm trying to lose weight. What else would I do there? Certainly not eat a cupcake." *You liar! You're lying about two things. Shame!*

"I want a vanilla cake with vanilla icing, and for flowers, let's go with roses." Dane continues to stare at the TV. "There, decided."

"I was hoping for something a little more elegant and tasty. And I'd prefer hydrangeas to roses."

"But vanilla is a safe flavor. Everyone likes it."

"Not everyone." My head's in a fog, and I blurt out, "Are you cheating on me?" I don't realize what I've asked until it's too late.

Dane chokes on his chicken and chugs his wine until it clears. "Why would you ask that?"

His question doesn't calm my racing thoughts. "Because you didn't answer your phone last night. What if I needed you? What if I had an emergency?" A lump rises in my throat, and I try my best to swallow it away.

"You have my desk phone number at the office." He sets his wine glass down. "Why didn't you call it?"

I feel the blood drain straight to my toes. "It completely slipped my mind. I'm sorry. It's just, we seem to be slipping away from each other, not together. We can't agree on wedding stuff or even make the time to discuss it."

"We did discuss it." Dane grabs my hand and cups it in his. I set my fork down and turn to him. Again, we're sitting on the couch for dinner, instead of at the kitchen table. And I realize how unromantic our dinners have become.

"Work's been insane lately. You know that. Plus, I'm trying to give you space so you can get to the gym. I want you to hit your goal. If you spend time with me every night, then when will you have time to work out?"

He has a point, not that I want to admit it, because it makes me look ridiculous for thinking he was unfaithful when I know that I've been having thoughts of Ed. *And lying about eating a cupcake*.

I sip my Cab to give myself a few seconds before I speak. "You're right. I mean after work it's already evening, fighting through traffic, letting Pear out, and heading to the gym. Most nights, I'm not eating until at least eight or nine."

Dane pauses the show on the TV, squeezes my hand, and lets it go. "See? Besides, in only a few short months we'll be living together. Relish the freedom because pretty soon you won't be able to get rid of me." He leans in and kisses my forehead.

I remember when he used to kiss me on the lips with passion, and now it's always just pecks here and there.

"Dane, we don't even know where we'll be living."

"Of course we do. Your house is too far from work for me, and ... it needs some repairs."

My eyes scan the room. Sure it could use a few upgrades, but it's cozy. *Why is it always his way over mine?*

"My house is closer to both our jobs, and it's up-to-date." He kisses my forehead again and returns to his plate. "You didn't think we'd live here, did you?"

His house is perfect if you like sterile and charmless. He hits play on his show as he stares off at the television like Pear staring at his favorite fetch ball. But as I watch Dane gaze at the actors on the screen, part of me wonders if he would've answered his work phone if I'd called it.

Chapter Seven

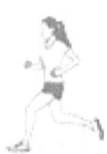

As I enter the gym the following night, my entire lower body, from my hips down, is stiff and sore. I'm wobbling from the pain like a robot.

I notice a shiny new sign on Eloise's desk, but she isn't working tonight. Instead, a man with gelled hair and two earrings in his left ear is at the desk. His name tag reads: Jaxtyn.

"Welcome," he cheers, as though my arrival is a royal occasion.

Because I'm exhausted from work, in tremendous pain, and I want to be anywhere but here, I allow my sarcasticness to flow.

"Thanks so much ... Jaxtyn. I'm delighted to be here. There's nothing I want to do more than to sweat my butt off on one of your fine machines." I bat my eyelashes as though they're a mile long.

He brings his hand to his chest, and his mouth falls open. "Well, that seems overdramatic."

I set my hand on the top of his desk and lean forward. "It's six-thirty on a weekday. I want nothing more than to be snuggled up on my couch with my dog, a glass of wine, and a trashy TV show, but instead, I'm here trying to lose weight, so I don't pop a seam on my wedding dress."

I start to walk away when I hear Jaxtyn shift in his chair and stand.

"If you're trying to lose weight, might I suggest laying off the vino," Jaxtyn calls after me.

I turn my head over my left shoulder. "You can, but that goes against your judgment-free zone rules, and I don't want to break another one of your signs."

The sound of Jaxtyn's gasp, followed by "You're her!" floats into the air.

I ignore him as I climb onto the treadmill, which in my current state looks like I'm trying to scale a fence. Wrapping my hand around the bar, I yank myself up onto the machine in one stiff lurching movement.

A part of me is glad Ed is not here. I'm not in the mood for any type of competition—and neither are my muscles. I only want to work out and go home. *Okay, I just want to go home. And not die. That would also be great. No death, please, especially on a treadmill, at my age.*

I'm five minutes into my choppy rhythm of walking-hobbling when Ed climbs onto the machine next to me.

I remove my left earbud and smile. "Hey, surprised to see you here—at the same time as yesterday."

My sarcasm is long-lasting today.

"I know, right?" he says, playing along.

My feet almost slide out from under me as I hold back a laugh and focus on my steps.

"Are you okay? You look like you're in pain?"

"Me? No." I wave off his comment. "I'm just a slight bit sore from yesterday. Means I'm doing it right."

"Don't push yourself if you're sore." He punches a few buttons on the machine, and it starts up. "Did you talk to Dane? Straighten everything out?"

I keep up my pace on the machine. "Yes, I think so, kinda. I mean, he reminded me I could've called his office phone." Saying the words aloud makes them seem not as sturdy as they have been for the last twenty-four hours. "But we didn't get anywhere with anything else." *I want a chocolate and caramel wedding cake.*

"Don't give up." Ed's muscles flex as he grabs hold of the bar. "I was going to see if you were up for a competition. Friendly, of course, but you need to be careful if you're hurting."

"I'm more than ready." I'm not, but I need the push to get me through the rest of this workout.

"Are you sure? You could hurt yourself if you overdo it."

"I'm sure." *I'm not.* When I woke up this morning, the cupcake I'd shared with Ed had done me zero favors. I had to lie down to get my work pants clasped. Halfway through the day, the imprint of the top button showed like a tattoo below my belly button. It was so tight I left it unbuttoned for the rest of the day. Thank goodness my long blouse covered up the front of my exposed underwear.

"If you're sure," Ed says. "Let's do ten minutes at a three percent incline."

I take a deep breath. The highest incline I've managed to get to is a sorry one percent incline. And even at that, I didn't last long before I needed to lower it back to a zero percent incline.

"Half the battle is in your mind, Hailey." Ed gazes at me the same way I look at a warm donut. "Don't overthink it."

"Okay, let's go." I punch it up to a three percent incline. *If legs can cry out in agony, mine just did.*

Ed jabs the air with his fist and lets out a cheer. I can't help but smile. He's such a dork, but not in a bad way.

At the end of ten minutes, I'm breathing hard but not dead. I can't believe I made it one minute at this incline, let alone a whole ten.

"Great job, Hailey!" Ed cheers. "Want to go another ten?"

"No, please, no," I gasp. My legs feel like they're walking through wet concrete.

Ed slows his machine down, and I do the same. "Let's call it a tie."

"No," I moan. "I don't want you to girl-it-up."

He chuckles. "Girl-it-up? Nice try, I'm not giving up that easy. We still have weights to lift." Ed jumps off the treadmill and puts his hands on his hips; like he's wearing a superhero cape and standing in front of a fan.

"We have what to what?" I hit the pause button on the machine and step off.

"You claim you don't want me to girl-it-up," Ed points at the stack of dumbbells across the gym, "so weights."

"Girls can lift weights. I can lift weights." Although I can't remember the last time I did. But my upper body is the only part that isn't sore. "Yes, weights, perfect."

I'm still out of breath a bit, but follow Ed to what might possibly lead me to a heart attack, or at least throw my back out.

He lifts two weights labeled twenty off the bar. I boldly reach for the ones labeled ten. As soon as they're in each hand, it takes everything I have to keep my chest from falling forward into the row of dumbbells.

"Whoa there, princess, those might be a bit heavy for you."

Princess? I'm as off-balance from the nickname as I am from the two weights threatening to rip my arms from their sockets.

I straighten my back. "I can handle ten pounds, no problem, but," I close my eyes and try to fight the strain, "I think I'll go with the five-pound ones instead."

In my attempt to gently set the weights back in their spot, I fail. They slip from my hands and drop with a clunk. I pick up the five-pound ones and control my facial expression of delight that I probably won't die now—at least not my upper body. My lower body is for sure a few seconds from death.

"Let's do two reps of fifteen," Ed declares.

I nod in agreement with the challenge. Yet, one rep in, and I'm pretty sure a vein in my neck and arms is going to explode.

"So," I huff, "What do you like to do for fun?"

Ed's biceps are straight in front of me, and I stare, a zone out type of stare. "I enjoy trying new restaurants and exploring new hiking trails. Does your fiancé workout?"

We hit fifteen, and I set the weights at my feet with a sigh. "Dane runs every morning. He's not big on gyms."

When I stretch my arms out, I notice something in my peripheral vision that I haven't seen before. *When did this happen?* I can't unsee the horrible sight, and I suddenly become religious. *Please, God, please don't let Ed see it too.*

Bat wings!

My arms have dangling wings. *Call the exterminator, we've got bats!*

Mental note: wear a long sleeve shirt when working out until I can lessen the visualization of *this* nightmare.

Ed motions for me to pick my two death sticks back up. "Why don't you run with him in the mornings? Spend more time together."

I turn slightly sideways in hopes that my wings become less noticeable. My breath is labored as I lift each weight into a butterfly curl. "First, I'm not a morning exercise person—or a morning person. Second, we don't live together, so one of us would have to drive to meet up for the run."

Hearing these excuses aloud makes me contemplate longer than I should that Dane and I don't sound like a great match, not to mention, an engaged couple.

"That's a shame," Ed huffs.

For some reason, I believe Ed is sincere in his statement, and I can't silently agree with him more. I don't mention the third reason why Dane and I never work out together. He likes to work out solo. Of course, I try not to be offended by this, but I am.

When Dane and I met, I had more time, more energy, and more desire to stay fit, but as work became more stressful and Dane and I spent more time together, working out fell to the wayside, or waist-side, actually. Some depression set in because I wanted to exercise with him and grow in our relationship. Since that was off the table, I spent my time alone, eating more than I should, and I became sedentary.

"Hey, everything okay?" Ed's voice breaks into my thoughts.

My eyes squint, disturbed by my feelings. "Yes, of course."

Chapter Eight

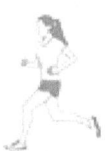

"The cake samples are here?" My mouth is watering before my bare feet reach the edge of Dane's living room rug. I'm hobbling a bit, but not as bad as yesterday.

"Yes, Cakes and More dropped off the samples a few hours ago."

My vision darts to Dane. "And you haven't stolen even one bite yet?"

"Of course not. I'm waiting for you." Dane has set up the mini cakes in the middle of the kitchen island.

Dane's kitchen is modern and sleek—white cabinets and white marble countertops. It's a kitchen meant for someone who doesn't spill cheap wine or spaghetti sauce, which is certainly not me.

He hands me a fork like it's the Olympic torch and kisses my forehead. "I can't wait for the big day. I'm ramping up my morning runs from three miles to four."

I resist the urge to roll my eyes as we lean against the island, not even bothering with the bar stools that sit against one side.

He pops open the lid of the first one. There are five distinct layers.

"This is peanut butter cup cake," Dane says, sticking his fork into it.

I'm way ahead of him and already have a bite in my mouth. I press the fork against my tongue as I pull it out. Chocolate and peanut butter mix with the chocolate frosting. "A bit too rich, I think."

Dane nods. "I think so too."

"What's next?" I'm already eyeing the next one.

"Vanilla Bean."

I'm hesitant as I slide the fork full of cake into my mouth. "Hey, not bad," I cover my mouth and mumble.

Dane shakes his head. "I think that's our winner."

"We still have three more to try." I point at the one with frosting that almost looks like they toasted it for a few minutes—tan on the white tips.

Dane slides over and pokes his fork into it. "Toasted vanilla."

We take a bite at the same time. Dane's eyes light up. Mine fizzle.

"I take it that's a no?" he asks.

I can barely swallow and shake my head.

He pushes a glass of water my way, and I take it, gulping it down. "It had an after-taste. I don't think the cake is supposed to have an after-taste."

Dane's face scrunches up. "Okay, that's a pass then."

"I'm ready for the next one." I move closer to Dane and the two final cake samples. "This one says party. What does that mean?"

Dane studies the label, as though I read it wrong. "Party?"

I lean closer, and my shoulder presses against Dane's arm. My nose catches a new cologne scent. "Do you think something is gonna explode out of it? Like a liquid center?"

Dane takes his fork and turns his face away as he pushes down into it. I live on the edge and remain within inches of it.

"Oh, it's a confetti cake!" I cheer and shove my fork into it.

"That's pretty good," Dane mumbles through the bite in his mouth.

I take my time, allowing my mouth to fully savor the cake and frosting. "Oh, yum." I point with my fork.

"Last one." Dane slides the chocolate frosted cake between us. "This one was a special request."

I look it over like an injured dog. "Special?"

"I hope you like it." Dane shoves his fork into it.

I do the same, and it's met with something sticky. As I take the bite, I realize it's chocolate and caramel. It's creamy and sticky, luxurious, and delicious.

"Divine," I say, once I finish the bite.

Dane's face does not register the same delight as mine.

"It's ..." He glances at me and then the cake. "It's okay, I guess."

"You think another one of the cakes is better?"

"The vanilla bean is the best one, followed by the party one. I wanted to try and give you the cake you wanted."

"But you aren't willing to allow me to have it because it's not your favorite?" *It's like dangling a ball on a string for a dog to chase but never to have.*

"We'll go with your cake then." He moves to throw away the leftover cakes. Saving them would apparently be unhealthy.

"Thanks?" I take another bite of the chocolate and caramel cake and wrap my hands around the container in an attempt to keep him from throwing it away. "I don't want to waste it."

Chapter Nine

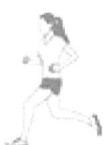

When I arrive at the gym two evenings later (I had no choice but to skip the gym until I could walk without looking like Herman Munster from my sore legs), I spot Ed already working out, but on the machine next to him is what I assume ... a model. Not one I recognize from a magazine, but one who could be in a magazine. Perfect hair, perfect figure. They're laughing, and she's not out of breath. I already don't like her.

I remind myself there's nothing to be jealous about because Ed and I are not dating—I mean because beauty is on the inside. I'm engaged to Dane. Ed and I are not even friends. We're only acquaintances. If the police ever question me, I wouldn't even be able to tell them Ed's last name.

I head to the treadmill at the end of the row, farthest away from Ed and the model. My legs are not one-hundred percent, and my arms are not feeling any stronger than mashed potatoes. *And now I'm hungry.*

I wrap my hand around the support bar and pull myself onto the machine. It's time to zone out. I slip my earbuds in, hit one percent incline, and start the sheer agony I'll face for an hour.

A few minutes in and show I'm watching on my phone is covered by a drop-down alert of an incoming video call. It's Dane.

If my face was not flushed already, it is now. The last thing I need is to look like a hot mess in front of my fiancé when I'm already worried about not being as sexy as I should—want to—be.

"Hey, Champion!" Ed startles me from behind.

My finger jets forward and swipes the phone's screen the opposite way of reject. Dane's face pops up onto it. In the commotion, I lose track of my feet and start to trip. Ed's strong hands reach for me. I feel them as they hold me upright around my waist.

In my earbuds, Dane says, "What's going on? Who's that?"

With one hand, Ed reaches around me and hits pause on the machine, but keeps his other hand on my waist. "Close call."

I glance at Ed's hand, and he instantly removes it from my midsection.

"Thanks," I whisper as though it's a secret.

Dane's voice is in my ear, "Hailey, what's going on?"

"Are you okay?" Ed asks, standing at the end of the treadmill.

"Yes, thank you." I turn to my phone and pick it up. "Sorry, Dane. I was working out. I'll call you back when I'm home." I hit END before he can respond.

I look around for the model.

"What are you doing way over here? Do I smell that bad?" Ed raises his arms and sniffs. "Not great, but not awful."

I chuckle, but I won't admit that I refuse to work out next to someone who looks like they live off five grapes and a coffee bean as their daily food intake.

"To be honest, I'm surprised to see you here." Ed runs a hand through his hair. "I figured you'd be sore for a lot longer after your workout extravaganza."

"I'm a bit sore—" *I'm still incredibly sore*, "but the calendar is catching up to me, plus with the upcoming holidays ..." *The food, the upcoming holiday food.*

"Well, I won't keep you, but don't overdo it, again. The last thing you need is to pull something and be out for a week." Ed backs up. "The weights are calling my name."

I nod and turn around. I hit start, focus on my steps, and return to the show I've been watching. Halfway through a text message from Mallory pops at the top of my phone's screen: **No news. It looks like your suspicions were just that, suspicions. Dane was working late.**

A sense of relief washes over me—at first, and then I wonder why I should have to worry about such a thing. But then I remember the new cologne I smelled on Dane. We aren't even married, and I'm already doubting all of it. Maybe he's not pulling away, perhaps I am.

My shoes press hard into the treadmill, and I feel the balls of my feet ache as I devise a plan to make it up to Dane. He always loves it when I make him blackened salmon over salad. What do I need to pick up at the grocery store? What do I have at home already? The rest of the gym blurs away as my excitement causes me to call Dane. But not a video call, because I'm aware I look like a glazed donut on fire. *And now I want a donut.*

"Hey, babe. I'm almost finished with my workout." I huff into the phone as I continue to power walk on the treadmill. "You're still coming over tonight, right?"

"What was going on earlier?"

"Oh, sorry about that, nothing important. So, I want to make you your favorite dinner."

"Sounds great. Let's have dinner at my place. When will you be over?"

I bite my lip. I can't take Pear with me to his place because Dane doesn't want fur on his precious rugs. (Another reason we don't live together yet.)

With being gone all day at work, I hate leaving Pear alone for the better part of the evening too. "I'm thinking maybe eight, but—"

"Great! Listen, I'll see you when you get here. I need to finish my crunches."

The call drops before I can request we stick with the plan to meet up at my place. I run my tongue over the front of my teeth and clamp my eyes shut with frustration for a second—poor Pear.

As I start my cool down, I catch something hot pink out of the corner of my eye. Turning my head, I spot a different model doing lunges in paradise pink high heels across the gym's open area.

My eyes squint in disbelief. "What the heck?"

"The ultimate workout." A woman says, appearing nearby the treadmill. Her hair is in such a high ponytail that it's practically on her forehead.

She nods her head the direction of the woman in heels and the ponytail bobs. "Supposed to help you tone your legs and more beneficial than wearing sneakers."

I continue to observe the miraculous miracle that's beauty and balance in one. Behind the woman in heels is Ed, but he seems to be the only one *not* checking her out. Instead, he's facing the wall of mirrors lifting a set of weights.

"Have you tried it before?" High-Ponytail elbows me.

"No." I shake my head, gazing at the fact that the woman's not even teetering a millimeter with each lunge.

After a few more seconds, I decide it's best to head home. I need to shower, apologize to Pear, and hit the grocery store on my way to Dane's place.

I catch my shoulders slumping. All I want to do is snuggle up on the couch after a nice long hot shower relaxes my sore muscles. It's not that I don't want to spend time with my fiancé, I do.

I must.

On the drive home, all I think about is the long day I had at work (including the kid who almost bit my finger off when I flossed his teeth). I check the time on my dash; it's already later than planned. Maybe I should call Dane and cancel, but I can't do that. We haven't seen each other much the last week.

It takes me ten minutes to shower, another ten to dress and throw on foundation, mascara, and lip gloss. Plus, five minutes to cuddle with Pear as I apologize for leaving him. But as I lock the front door I hear Pear whimper and tears form at the edges of my eyes.

How will Dane live full time with a dog? And what about getting another dog, something I've mentioned several times. About a year into our relationship, we started discussing kids, and when we'll want to have them, but never dogs.

It's nearly eight-thirty when my pointer finger pushes the doorbell at Dane's house. *Do the neighbors notice me out here—ringing the doorbell instead of having a key?* It showcases that his home is one hundred percent his and not, now or possibly ever, ours.

The weight from the grocery bags in my hand pulls my arm down as though it's holding the weight of my thoughts.

Dane swings the door open. "Hey, babe." He steps aside as I enter. "I'm starving. I squeezed an extra workout in tonight."

After removing my shoes, I make my way to the back end of the house and heave the bags onto the kitchen counter.

"You're okay having Pear with us after we get married?" I blurt out. "And we can adopt more dogs, too, right?"

He starts to dig through the grocery bags. "Yeah, we can discuss that later. No rush. What are you making? You said it's my favorite, but I have a few."

"Dane, this is important." A lump in my throat that I don't expect causes me to choke on my words. "We can't keep putting everything off."

His hand touches my back. "Sure, Pear can live with us as long as he stays on the floor. He'll only be allowed in the kitchen and living room. But another dog? I think one's plenty. They shed and drool on everything."

"Pear sleeps with me in bed every night, and we cuddle on the couch." My forehead creases as I press my palms into the countertop. "I can't go changing up what he's used to."

Dane's hand grazes my shoulder. "He'll learn to be more independent." He kisses my forehead.

"I don't want him more independent. He's my baby. You make it sound like he's an unwelcome guest." I reach for the cupboard and pull out a frying pan. The kiss his lips left starts to feel like a burn.

"I said we can keep Pear. I know he's your dog. But we need to focus on our family. Our future." Dane kisses my forehead again and heads to the living room, easing into his black leather couch.

As I prepare the meal, I fight back my tears. Our relationship is sitting on a fault line, and I sense an earthquake coming.

Chapter Ten

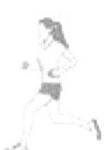

"**B**abe." Dane is behind me and puts his hands on my shoulders. "Are you crying?"

I wipe a tear off my cheek with the back of my hand.

"Hold on, what's up?" Dane's fingers press into my shoulders.

"Pear means everything to me. And I want more dogs. I guess I ... I thought things would be different over time. I thought you'd grow to love him." I lean my head back and try to prevent the remaining tears from falling.

"Come here, let's talk." Dane reaches for my hand.

"But dinner?" I mumble.

He leads me to the couch; my hands are still damp from washing the greens. As Dane sits, I follow as we face each other, our knees touching.

"Babe, I know you love Pear. I would never ask or expect you to give him up." He runs his hand on my leg. "I think that another dog, down the road, can be discussed, but I want to have some time for us, and then to have kids."

I glance down at his hands. "Don't you love Pear?"

"I love you, and that's what matters. Pear is your dog, and he's a good dog."

Dane's words or lack of feelings, slice me open like a cantaloupe. How could I be so freaking blind?

"But if having another dog will make you happy then ... we can."

This is not what I want to hear, in that tone. It's not us, but him and I.

"It would make me happy, but I want it to make us happy." Maybe I'm overreacting to his non-love for Pear. After all, he is my dog. Perhaps if we get a puppy together it'll be different.

"We'll be happy. There'll be rules. Not on the furniture, in the crate whenever we're gone. And it won't prevent us from doing everything we want to do."

As Dane's words to sink in, I remind myself that my way is not the only way to think. Just because I consider dogs to be family, it doesn't mean that others have to do the same—but they should.

"So, we're okay." Dane squeezes my hand. "I love you, and I want you to be my wife more than anything in the world."

My teeth pull in my lower lip. "I can't wait to be your wife."

Yet, something twitches inside. And I know I'm confused as to what I'm feeling. I pray it's cold feet about the newness that comes with a pending marriage. I have a history of being engaged and calling it off—twice. I'm not going to do it again. Not this time. I'll be thirty this year, and my eggs are probably starting to dry up like old grapes on the vine. Life is not going to wait for me. *So, stop making excuses.*

Dane leans forward, his lips brush mine long enough for me to pull myself from my thoughts. As we part, he says, "Love you, babe."

"Love you, too." I stand. "I'm going to finish getting dinner ready."

He snatches up the remote and changes the channel as I make my way back into the kitchen.

About an hour later, I serve our dinner on his coffee table in front of the couch.

"Looks great, but bread?" Dane takes his plate and moves it closer to him.

I nod. Yes, I cut us a few small pieces off a baguette to have with the meal. Apparently, I shouldn't have done this. *This is getting to be too much, even for me.*

"How's your weight loss goal coming?" He eyes the bread on my plate as though I'm a child who's storing my gum there.

"Great," I lie and tear off a chunk of bread. "I'm going to wear heels to the gym tomorrow."

Chapter Eleven

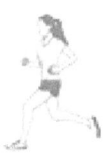

I do a slow circle inside the for-sale condo. Everything is shiny and bright, from the creamiest-tan tile to the beige walls, and the floor-to-ceiling windows. *I hate it all.*

"It's perfect," Dane says, his hands are inside his pockets, pushing back his sports jacket. "See, Hailey, compromise. Not my place or yours."

My face contorts. It's far from perfect.

"Hailey?"

I turn to Dane. "It's definitely glamorous, but I'm not sure it's my style."

"That's what's great. We can make it our style. It solves which house to pick—a collaborative start."

"It doesn't have a yard for Pear."

Dane's hand moves to his chin. "It has a little dog area downstairs where you can take him out to use the restroom."

"He needs more than an area." I walk up to the window in the living room and look out at the Estrella Mountains in the distance. "I know you're excited about this place. The view is amazing, but it's not the best fit for us. Do you really want to raise a family here? Without a yard or room to grow?"

"There's a great park across the street, lots of palm tree-lined paths." Dane crosses his arms.

"It's just not what I envisioned if we sold our places and got something together." I glance at him.

"Marriage is about compromise." He reaches for my hand, and our fingers lock together.

While I know marriages, *all* relationships, are about compromises, maybe this is too far a stretch for me. Not to mention one-sided. This condo is one-hundred percent ("Dane fabulous"). It's not about compromising on wallpaper patterns, or if we have chili or soup for dinner. Where we live is huge.

I pull my phone from my back pocket.

"I should go." I step toward the door. "Need to work out."

When I open the condo's front door, the real estate agent is waiting in the hall, her thumb is scrolling on her cell phone. "So, is the happy couple ready to make an offer?"

A weak smile creases my lips. "Thank you for showing us this place. It's nice, but not what I'm looking for."

I realize I refer to "us" as "I" and my heart clutches in my chest. "I mean what *we're* looking for, for us. I have a dog, and he needs a yard."

The agent slides her phone into her purse as Dane exits the condo, stopping behind me.

"We'll revisit this later tonight." Dane puts his hand on my shoulder, the weight of it is as heavy as a brick.

I turn and kiss him on the cheek. "I'll leave you two to discuss dog-friendly options." I wiggle from beneath Dane's hand and scurry down the hall.

When I reach my car, the sound of my heart pounds in my ears, and my face is flushed. My hands instinctively find the steering wheel and I grip it noticing I'm breathing like I just ran a marathon. Not that I know what that feels like, but I know what mild running is like, and I suck at it, and this is far worse.

I fumble with my cell but manage to call Mallory. Thankfully, she picks up on the third ring.

"Hey, Hailey."

"Hi," I say half-gasping.

"You don't sound good, are you okay?"

I shake my head 'no.' "I hope this is cold feet."

"What's cold feet? Do you want to meet up?"

I lean my head back on the seat and let my left hand slide from the steering wheel. "Dane had me meet up with him at this condo with his real estate agent. I didn't even know he had an agent, let alone was looking for a place for us. And a condo. *A condo*!"

"That's a good thing. You won't have to decide who sells what."

"Did you hear me? *Con-do*. I don't want to live in a condo. I want a house. A nice big house with a huge yard."

There's pressure in my throat from the lump forming, holding back whatever emotions I'm trying to desperately ignore.

"Honey, just tell Dane. Keep looking. There's still time before the wedding."

"I ... I need to go workout. I can't deal with this right now."

"Hailey, are you going to work out because you want to lose weight?"

"What? Of course, that's the whole point."

"What I mean is, are you working out for you? Or are you sure you're not running away towards something else, something new?"

"That's ridiculous." But as I end the call with Mallory, I'm not sure of anything.

Chapter Twelve

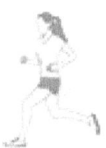

E loise eyes me over the top of her cell phone when my
high heels tap past her.

Since I rarely wear heels, I'm sure I'll have some sore feet
later. However, I do my best to shake off the feeling as I step
up onto the treadmill.

I don't see Ed—or the models—anywhere, and I already
feel more confident. Maybe there's something behind heels
and working out.

The first few minutes I take it slow and hold onto the treadmill bars. The coordination it takes to walk on the machine
with the heels requires extra concentration, but it gets easier
once I get the rhythm down.

Soon, my calves burn like hot sauce in the eye. I'm finally
able to let go of the bars as sweat forms in all the places it
should—and shouldn't. *Like behind my chubby knees.*

"What are you doing?" Ed's voice startles me.

My hands jet out and grab the sidebars to keep upright. "I'm
working out. What are you doing?"

Ed punches the buttons on the machine next to me and begins to jog. He sets his phone up on the ledge. "I'm about to listen to the best mix of songs ever created," he eyes me, "and wait for you to trip and fall."

"I won't be tripping or falling." I let go of the bars and tap the arrow on the incline setting up one. *That's right, two percent incline!* "And I doubt you have the best music mix."

Ed's smile is visible from the side, and I find myself smiling with him. He's piqued my interest. "Can I listen to it?"

He hands me one of his blue-tooth earbuds, and I reach out to take it while straining to keep myself upright.

A part of me is nervous because I have no idea what type of music to expect. By looking at Ed, I would guess either indie rock or techno. Dane's favorite music is jazz and classical, but it doesn't take any skill to look at him for half a second and guess that.

A song starts, and my mouth opens wide as I turn to him. "Is this '90s music? *You* like '90s music?" I squawk.

He chuckles, "Yes, I take it you're surprised?"

"No, it's just, well ..." I struggle to maintain my pace on the treadmill while trying to process this excellent discovery about Ed. "Okay, yeah, I'm surprised." I blush.

"We both seem to be kids of the '90s, so it makes sense from that regard."

"Are you claiming to know how old I am?" I place my hand on my chest, my fingers outstretched.

"Age smage. Your real age is your soul. And your soul is whatever age you make it."

My breath catches as I soak in his beautiful words. Learning Ed's point of view is a refreshing and welcome change in my life. With Dane, age matters, and status matters. And I have no idea where happiness falls.

The next song is by the Spin Doctors, and the beat of the drums vibrates through me. "I haven't heard this song in forever."

"The best workout soundtrack ever made." Ed narrows his eyes. "Let me guess, you love country music or country-pop music."

"It's not a good idea to assume." I wag my finger at him.

"But I'm right."

"Okay," I roll my eyes, "you're correct. Let me guess, you loved shows like *Baywatch* and *MacGyver*."

"So did you!" he declares.

I fight off a smile by biting the inside of my cheek. "Those were good shows!"

"They don't make them like they used to. Everything now is reality, reality, reality."

"Hey, those are my guilty pleasure shows. Plus, they have been rebooting some of them."

"It's not the same rebooted. So, how long do you plan on working out in heels?"

I glance down. "As long as I need to to hit my goal."

He gazes at me in a parental look, as though he's trying to decide if I've eaten enough green beans to be excused from the dining table.

"What?" My hand, palm up, jets his direction. "If the model does it, then it must work."

"Model? What model?"

I wave him off.

"How about you do what you want to do and be who you want to be," Ed says.

"I want to look attractive, especially in my wedding dress." I'm so frustrated with how I feel I'm trying not to cry.

"Maybe you already do." He shakes his head.

For a moment, I don't realize what Ed said, and blurt out, "There is no way I can walk down the aisle looking like this." Then his words catch up to me. "Wait. What?"

"I don't want to cross any lines, but stop pushing yourself to be a specific someone for someone else and be what's best for you. Working out should be for being healthy, not to try and look like Miss All-I-Eat-Are-Salads."

"You mean to tell me that you don't want a perfect woman on your arm? Of course, you do."

"What I mean is, do what matters to you. Don't lose yourself by focusing on wanting to lose weight for your fiancé or a wear-it-once-dress. Nothing else matters but you and your health. And if that's all your fiancé cares about, then ... I'm sorry."

My right foot cramps up as his words roll through one ear while the music blasting from the earbud vibrates the other. I reach for the bars, but I'm too late.

"Going down!" I scream.

One heel goes flying as I crash and catapult off the end of the treadmill. The tread rubs against my arm like sandpaper, scratching the bare skin, and I lean backward to prevent it from doing any more damage.

Ed lunges for my machine and shuts it off with a slap of his palm. He drops to the floor next to me.

"Don't move," he instructs as his eyes scan me over. "Does anything feel broken?"

I shiver, feeling Ed's vision inspecting me. It feels so personal, so deep. Tears form on the bottoms of my eyelids.

"I can't do this," I blubber. "I'm so tired of being fat and ugly. Nothing is working."

"Don't you dare say that." As his hand touches my knee, I flinch. I'm wearing jogger sweatpants, so I have no idea what's happened to my legs underneath it.

"It's the truth!" I wipe my tears with the back of my hand. "I just want to be beautiful. I want to be strong. I'm so tired of hating myself."

Ed takes my arm at my elbow; blood is forming at the scratch. "Don't hate yourself. I sure don't."

With Ed close, I'm aware of his scent. He smells like grass after the rain. Every part of me wants to lean closer to him, and I do. Breathing Ed in is comforting, like a warm from the dryer blanket on a rare rainy day in Phoenix.

I don't know how long I've been gazing off as the tears continue falling ... until faster than an egg cracking, I'm back to reality with several burns radiating through my skin.

"Can you stand up?" he asks.

"Of course," I fib and ease myself up with Ed's help. With his support, I hobble over to a nearby empty bench. I have one heel on and no idea where the other one flew off to.

"I'm going to get some first aid supplies and take care of your arm." Ed springs away like he has air-filled pump-up '90s sneakers on and heads over to the front desk. He returns with a small white box and sets it between us.

"Thank you, but I can clean myself up. I have no idea how banged up my knees are under here."

"Let me take care of your arm first." Ed sprays on some antiseptic, and I wince. "Sorry."

He glances up at me, and I'm instantly infatuated. There are speckles of amber in his brown eyes.

"It's okay," I whisper.

He wraps the gauze around my arm. "Are you alright?"

Somehow I know he's not only asking about my visible injuries. "Sorry, I let my emotions get the best of me."

"Don't apologize." Ed's still holding my arm, and his fingers are gentle against my skin. "Are you sure you're okay to drive? Will your fiancé be there when you get home?"

I shake my head, no. "My dog, Pear, he's pretty good at taking care of me." I smile at the thought of him.

"Dogs are the best." Ed lets go of my arm, and I instantly feel weak.

"So, you like dogs?" I ease myself to stand.

"Like would be a poor word choice." Ed stands next to me, looking me over like I'm a thick and juicy steak. "I love dogs. I have three at home waiting for me to finish up here."

I bite my lip. Of course he does.

Chapter Thirteen

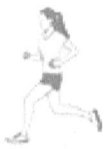

D ane sits next to me on the couch while I text Mallory photos of my scraped up knees and elbow.

"You think you'll be able to work out tomorrow? Or will you have to hold off a day?" Dane glances at me like I have a paper cut. "I'd be able to push through the pain."

"Seeing as though it burns just looking at it, no, I think I'll have to skip a day," I snap.

Dane's hand flexes around the remote. "Sorry, I was trying to make sure you were on track for your goal. You don't have to be defensive. I want the best for you."

What I want to say to Dane ("You're being rude") and what I'm about to say to Dane are two different things. "Thanks."

The reason why I don't say anything is because I shouldn't have to tell him how he should be. I don't want to spend my life wishing and hoping for Dane to be the way I want him to be. I can't change him. Once I start acting like his mother, I can't undo it. I refuse to be his mother. He already has one.

Mallory had gone down the path of nagging wife with Jack. For them, it works, but I refuse to give Dane excuses and nag him. There's no point in doing that. I want a man who is one hundred percent himself. I also want him to be one hundred percent willing to love me and be my partner because he wants to, not because I'm driving him nuts, and he just wants me to be quiet.

My stomach growls. "I should make dinner." I move to stand and peek at Dane.

"Oh, did you want me to help with that? I should, right?" He scurries to stand. "Do you have green beans or broccoli? I can do some steamed veggies and brown rice."

"For dinner or an appetizer?" I cross my arms and press my lips together in a firm line.

"For dinner, of course." Dane pauses mid-way into the kitchen. "Did I say something wrong? You've been moody lately." He chuckles. "Talk about being a bridezilla."

I'm not laughing. Maybe it's the horrific burn on my aching knees. Maybe it's the four aspirin. Maybe it's the truth setting itself free, but I can't hold my tongue. "What's with the new cologne? Why don't you like the way I look anymore? What changed?" *Besides my weight. Don't you dare say weight.*

My metal strainer crashes on the counter. I watch Dane from the couch attempt to wrap his hands around it to silence it. It's wobbling like a dreidel about to tip over.

"I didn't know I needed to check with you before I bought cologne. And, of course, I still love you, Hailey."

"You *still* love me?" I lean forward. "As though it's a chore?"

"Is it *that* time of the month? Not that I need to know, but this is very out of character for you."

My eyes grow wide in anger. "Excuse me. What the heck, Dane? Do you have an issue with the fact that I'm not as perfectly proportioned as I was when we met? Do you have an issue with my stomach spilling over my pants?"

Dane freezes like he's in the middle of a hold-up. "You're acting like going to the gym and eating healthy is hard. It's not."

"Stop bringing that up. I'm sick of hearing it."

"You're making it harder than it needs to be."

I move my tongue over the front of my teeth, trying to fight off the hurt that's welling up in my throat. It feels like I'm holding back vomit. Dane's "I still love you" is not "I love you," but a cover-up of the fact that he doesn't love me the same as he once did when I was eye candy on his arm. Now, I'm a big stuffed cookie, and while some might find me sweet, he doesn't anymore.

"Hailey, I do love you." Dane sits next to me on the couch, my non-leather, creamy plush slip-covered couch. "But ... "

Pear is curled up next to me between the plump pillows with "Happiness is a Dog" and "Fur-Loved" stitched on them.

"But ..." I coax him.

Dane takes my hand. "I don't see why it's hard for you to lose a little weight. I've managed to maintain my body by stepping up my workouts. Honestly, I thought the upcoming wedding would entice you."

The room turns fuzzy before my eyes. The temperature spikes within me and I'm hot. Too hot. I pull my hand away from Dane and hold it close to my chest. "I won't be your perfect woman, Dane."

"I'm not asking you to be perfect. I'm asking you to be what you were."

"Get out," I whimper. The tears are making my vision even fuzzier.

"Hailey, stop." His hand brushes my shoulder, and his once welcome touch feels like tiny push pins against it. "You're just having pre-wedding jitters, which is perfectly normal. Remember you've called off weddings before. Let me finish cooking dinner."

"Get out," I say louder this time.

"You're overreacting. I'm being honest with you because I love you. I'm marrying you, aren't I?"

Oh my goodness, aren't I? I ease myself off the couch and pinch my eyes closed in pain as I make my way to the door. Pear remains on the couch, but he's awake now and in alert mode.

I swing open the door as the cool fall air tickles my wet cheeks. "Get out of my house!" I choke over the lump in my throat.

Dane snatches his car keys off the entryway table. "Call me when you're feeling better."

As he leans in to kiss my cheek, I pull back. The back of my head touches the door.

"Hailey." He reaches out for my hand.

But instead of letting him take my hand in his, I take his wrist and turn his hand over, so his palm is up. I set the engagement ring in it. "Goodbye, Dane."

He stumbles backward, staring at his hand. When I close the door, the last thing I see is the sadness in Dane's eyes. And no doubt it will haunt me in my sleep tonight.

Chapter Fourteen

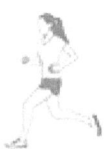

M allory squeezes a slice of lemon into her iced tea. We sit opposite each other in the chestnut-colored booth at our favorite mom and pop restaurant, Mercers. The crowd of snowbirds dispersed about twenty minutes ago, allowing several of the televisions on the wall to be heard again.

"Do you want to tell me what happened?" Mallory takes another bite of her turkey burger.

"Does it matter at this point?" I wiggle my ring finger at her. "We're no longer engaged."

"A relationship doesn't end by giving back a ring. In fact, I think most keep the ring or at least throw it out a car window while going over a bridge."

"This is Arizona; we don't have a lot of bridges." I bite into a fry. The grease and salt on my tongue has been missed.

"Lots of couples call off weddings for one reason or another, and it doesn't mean the relationship is over. This is not your first rodeo. You and Dane had a disagreement."

"Do you honestly think Dane and I are a good couple?"

Mallory looks over my shoulder at the television and bites the sides of her mouth, sucking in her cheeks. She makes eye contact with me. "I honestly thought you would be together for the long haul."

My eyes wrinkle up. "You compared us to a road-trip?"

Mallory shakes her head. "Ha, ha, no. I thought you two might get married and make a beautiful family someday, but things changed. For you both. You'd just gotten out of another relationship back when you met Dane."

I point a fry at her. "Call it what it was: another broken engagement."

"Doesn't matter, lots of people break off engagements, cheaper than a divorce."

I nod and take a sip of ice water. I've only cried once since the breakup. And it causes a guilty feeling in my heart because I should be more broken up about it.

"Anyway, both of you changed. You figured out more about yourself, and sadly, we see that Dane started to show his true colors. Sometimes colors take a while to show up. Or as you unwrap the rubber band around a person, the colors show."

"Tie-dye."

Mallory nods. "Tie-dye."

"Maybe Dane's right, I mean, I'm at fault for not looking the same."

"Oh please, do you think I look the same under my clothes? I've had twins. Jack and I have grown together. You and Dane grew, but not in the same direction. Jack and I have disagreements and arguments, but nothing that isn't fixable. Our biggest argument is who forgot to put the clothes in the dryer, or if we want to eat at the restaurant or get a to-go order. You and Dane disagreed on big things."

"Why didn't I see it?"

"Because you wanted it to work. You loved him." Her eyes narrow, "Love him?"

"I do love him, but I'm not in love with him, not anymore, seeing all of our big disagreements, our different ways of how we live life."

"And was it about the weight loss?"

I push the ice around in my glass with my straw. "It was about so much more than the weight. It was about Pear and our lifestyles and, ultimately, our goals and dreams. I love dogs and shabby chic decor. He likes straight edges and fish. Plus, I can't live my life scared about my weight. What if I have a baby and didn't lose the weight? What if I have a stroke, and only half of my body works?"

"You'd have a stroke just living in fear of having a stroke."

I nod my head in agreement.

"Dane hasn't always been that way, has he?" Mallory leans back into the booth.

"I think maybe he always has, but I didn't give much attention to his likes and dislikes until they were a problem." I take a fry and fold it into my mouth. "I think what you're saying is that by gaining weight, I actually saved myself a huge mistake."

"Yes, so much so that we should probably split a chocolate milkshake, just to be sure that you are back to your senses."

Chapter Fifteen

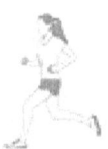

E loise gives me a half-smile as I enter the gym after a three-day absence. My knees are feeling a lot better, and I can walk without my facial expression looking like someone is giving me a spanking.

I arrive at the gym right before the after-dinner rush. It's mostly vacant, and I select the middle treadmill. It feels like having a movie theater all to myself.

I punch in a one percent incline and remind myself I'm now here to work out for me, for my health, and not to fit into a specific outfit for a particular person. Surprisingly, this makes my desire to work out not as much of a chore. A smile warms my face.

I'm in a good jogging rhythm when my nose alerts me to Ed before my vision does. A part of me has missed his scent, and I didn't even know it.

"Great to see you, Hailey." Ed hops onto the machine next to me. "Are your knees better?"

"Hey, thanks. Yes, a lot better. Not one hundred percent, but I'm not going to push myself too hard, yet."

"I'm just glad to see you decided on appropriate gym shoes." He eyes my sneakers.

"It was pretty stupid of me to work out in heels."

"We're all allowed to make mistakes." He sets his towel on the arm bar. "I'm just glad you're okay."

"Thanks." I bite my lip to keep from grinning too much.

Ed slips in his earbuds, and I return to the show on my cell phone. I relish in the happiness of walking next to him. For the first time in my weight loss journey I'm enjoying my workout. Maybe this is why people like going to the gym, on their own accord, for their own reasons.

"Why do you look so happy?" Ed asks as I step off the treadmill some forty-five minutes later. "Nothing wrong with it, of course, but usually you look like someone is holding you at gunpoint when you work out."

"I did? I do?" I wipe the sweat off my brow with my small gray towel.

"Yes, I'm guessing you're excited about your wedding."

Before I can answer him, Dane walks into the gym. He spots me and hurries over.

"Mallory said you'd be here." Dane's wearing workout clothes, but I don't know why, it's not the morning. "You haven't returned any of my voicemails or texts."

Ed runs his hand through his hair. "I think I'm going to hit the weights."

"Make sure they don't hit you back," I joke. And it's such a lame one I smack my hand to my forehead.

Ed finger guns me and hurries toward the rack of weights. Super lame, but delightfully cute too.

"Dane, I'm not ready to speak with you. Excuse me, I need to lift weights." I hurry off towards Ed.

Dane scurries behind me like a toddler.

I pick up two five-pound dumbbells and start to do bicep curls. Dane positions himself between Ed and me, although Ed is at least ten feet away and has spun around, so his back is to us.

"I'm sorry about the weight stuff, the dinner stuff, and Pear. Look, I'm here to work out, in a gym, with other people, at night." Dane waves his hand around as if I don't know where here is. "And Pear can sit on the couch."

I pause mid-curl. "It's okay, Dane, you shouldn't have to compromise with what you want, and I shouldn't either."

"Would it make you feel better if we moved the wedding date from Valentine's Day to sometime in March?"

I tilt my head like Pear does when I ask him if he wants to play fetch. "Feel better? Because I'd have more time to lose weight?"

"Yes." Dane grins. And then his face realizes like a bolt of lightning that that was the wrong answer. He shakes his head. "No, no, that's not what I meant. Hailey, please."

He drops to one knee and looks up at me with puppy eyes. "I'm sorry. I don't know what I'm saying. I'm trying to make it right."

"Get up, Dane." I lower the weights back onto the rack and shake out my hands. "Don't be sorry. You can't make it right."

"I don't understand." Dane stands.

"I don't either," Ed says from behind Dane.

"You're not helping," I tell Ed.

His face contorts. "Sorry, it's a habit to step in."

I cross my arms over my chest. "Dane, I want you to be with the woman of your dreams. And that's not me."

"It's not you?" Ed croaks.

"Oh my gosh." My fists clench.

"Sorry, sorry." Ed scurries past me and toward the bench press area, out of earshot of Dane and me.

"Come here." I grab Dane by the hand and pull him towards the lobby of the gym. Once we're in the small space, I notice Eloise standing and leaning over her desk.

I spin Dane around to face the door, and push him outside. The sun has set, filtering the sky with orange and pink shades over the parking lot. I place my hands on Dane's shoulders as he sulks. "You know we aren't a great match. Maybe we were when we first started dating, but I think both of us know, always knew, it wasn't meant to be. We changed. We grew."

"But I want to change. I will grow."

I shake my head. "No, even if you do, it's not you. You won't be happy in the long run, and I don't want to marry you only to get divorced."

Dane looks out at the sky. "How can it be so beautiful out in a moment like this?" He takes my hand, and I allow him to. "I don't want you to hate me."

I squeeze his hand. "I don't hate you. I want you to be honest with yourself. I think you're a jerk for how you treated me."

He presses his lips together. "I don't think it was about the weight. Focusing on it might've been because I saw issues within our relationship."

"Maybe you thought ... maybe *we* thought, if I lost the weight, it would fix all the issues we *weren't* talking about."

"I don't deserve you, Hailey." Dane lets go of my hand.

"You're right." *You don't.* I sigh. "I watched some romance movies over the last few days, and I realized I should pack up the things you had at my house and bring them back to you."

"I don't think I left anything there."

"Exactly. And there's nothing of mine at your place after *two* years. We should've seen this a long time ago."

Dane hugs me, and a part of me doesn't want it to end, because when it does, I have to face the fact that I've had another broken engagement.

We part, and he kisses me on the cheek. When I turn around, Ed's inability to hide behind a pole causes me to laugh. Without a doubt, he's been watching the entire time.

I head inside, past Eloise, who appears as confused as a city girl in the country. "So *that* was your fiancé?" she points at the parking lot.

I nod my head. "Yeah, why?" I wait for her to say something stupid.

"So he's, like, single now?"

I lean towards her desk. "He's all yours, honey. Let me know if you want his number." I slap the desk with the palm of my hand as Eloise jumps and reaches for the **JUDGMENT-FREE ZONE** sign.

I continue to the weight area and find Ed trying to appear as though he's been busy with a workout this entire time. I pick the five-pound dumbbells back up.

"Everything okay?" Ed asks without looking at me.

"For once, I do believe it is."

"So, the wedding is off?"

"The relationship is off." I do tricep extensions. *Dang those bat wings. They will disappear.* "I don't know if I'll ever get back to the shape I want to be in, but that's okay. I'll be happy, and that's what matters."

My triceps burn, and I push through it. "I'll marry the right man someday, and it'll be for all the right reasons."

"I have no doubt." Ed moves to the bench press. "Do you think Pear might enjoy a play date?"

"Of course, oh yes, because you have dogs."

You know, at the end of one of those television shows from the '90s, where two people look at each other with intense joy and smile just as they pause and run the credits over it ...

"Mini, Mighty, and Mo. They're great dogs," he mentions.

Ed and I are having *that* moment, and I know I'll remember it for the rest of my happy life.

Forty Before the New Year
(Enjoy this bonus novella!!)

by Savannah Hendricks

Originally published in the *Kissing at Midnight* a sweet romance anthology from <u>Literary Crush Publishing (2019)</u> and edited by Arielle Bailey.

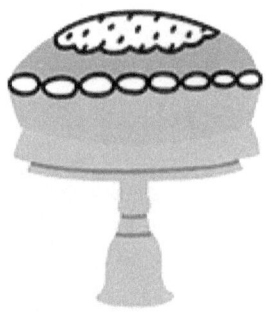

One

"**I** can do this." Maribelle sighed and snatched yet another magazine from the stack on the coffee table.

"I want to support you." Bridget shifted in her spot on the plush linen white couch. "But you had an entire year to make everything, and now you want to knock it out in a week?"

"You're the prime example of how *not* to be a best friend." Maribelle over-dramatically flipped her elbow-length golden blonde hair with her hand.

Bridget pressed her lips together. "Hmm, hmm."

The sheer floral blue and white curtains filtered the morning sunlight across the living room floor of Maribelle's studio apartment in Charleston. Even on her teacher's salary, she'd managed to decorate it in the chicest of southern charm decor, thanks to weekend trips to the flea markets.

She reached for the paper to-go cup containing her latte and took a long sip. "Thanks for stopping and getting breakfast." Maribelle eyed the empty bag of beignets with grease stains on the bottom and sides.

"My pleasure." Bridget rested her head on the velvety lilac pillows surrounding her on the couch. "This is your winter break; let's do something fun." She twisted a strand of auburn curl around her pointer finger. "Let's set you up on a date."

"No." Maribelle sprung up from the couch, the *Southern Living* magazine in her hand, waving it around like a flag. "Did you miss all of this flawed year?" She paced the living room floor; her vision on her Christmas red painted toenails.

"I know you've had a few break-ups," Bridget whined.

"A few?" Maribelle returned to the couch and tucked her legs under her as she sat down. "It felt like I had twenty break-ups."

Bridget stretched out her hand and wrapped it around Maribelle's shoulder. "Jason and Kurt were bad break-ups, I know, it felt like a lot more."

Maribelle shook her head and gazed at the many stacks of *Southern Living* magazines dating back to the first one released in 1966. Her grandma had collected each one and stored them in a corner hutch located in her dining room just off the kitchen. The issues stopped in the early two-thousands when Grams moved into the nursing home in Summerville. When Maribelle's parents sold Gram's house, she inherited the prized magazines, along with the hutch and all her bakeware.

She glanced over at it, nestled between the Christmas tree and the fireplace. The seafoam green had chipped and peeled over the years. However, Maribelle liked it looking a bit beat up because it held charm. Her Grams, unlike the hutch, had been far from flawed, and closer to perfect. But, Maribelle hoped that maybe she could at least make something from nothing if the cooking and baking skills would transfer from the magazines right through her fingertips.

"I know you want to honor your Grams and follow through on your New Year's promise to her, but will she know if you don't?" Bridget brought her coffee cup to her mouth, and all Maribelle could see was a pile of curls and two ocean blue eyes.

"Of course, Grams will know!" Maribelle asserted. "This is South Carolina. Her ghost is probably enjoying some hot tea in my kitchen right this minute." Maribelle's eyes darted toward the kitchen and back at Bridget.

Maribelle shook her head at her best friend's naïve ways. Bridget had moved here after college and knew nothing of southern culture, being from California. They'd met through mutual friends at a book club meeting held at the Charleston library, and bonded over the last two years. However, now that Bridget was engaged, they spent less and less time together. Maribelle knew their once-weekly breakfasts, and once-monthly dinners would likely be a thing of the past before too long. Everyone was finding love, but her.

"I promised Grams, and I'm keeping my word." Maribelle swallowed, as she took in the stacks of magazines about to tumble over. Her thoughts turned to Grams, saying goodbye to her last December. She never went back on her word. "I only need to make one recipe from each year."

"You have six days."

"I know." Maribelle frowned.

Bridget held up her hand, and tapped her fingers together, no doubt counting in her head. "That's forty recipes. Forty, not four."

"That puts me at about six and a half recipes a day." Maribelle bit her lower lip and her shoulders slouched. She took her hair and messily piled it at the top of her head, securing it with a clip from the end table. "It's a lot of recipes, but it's not like the world treats me well outside of this apartment. Staying inside to knock out all the cooking and baking might be just what I need to finish the year off right. Yet, if this year is any indication of next year, I'm not leaving my apartment come January first."

"You don't leave your apartment much anymore."

"I leave it every Monday through Friday for work. It just seems like whenever I'm out in the world, all I want to do is hide from it. There's a lot of love going on in Charleston. And I'm not a part of it." Maribelle observed her Christmas décorations throughout the living room and what spilled into the kitchen. She'd overdone it for sure, but with so much time procrastinating and crying over men, what else was she supposed to do?

"What'll you do with all the food?" Bridget traded magazines.

Maribelle's eyes lit up. How'd she not thought of this when she made the New Year's goal in the first place? "I'm going to do what Grams did, donate the meals to the church to serve for their daily lunches."

The church, as white as a wedding gown, sat at the corner of Magnolia and Main. They'd provided free lunches seven days a week for the homeless, no questions asked, for centuries.

Residents were encouraged to drop off donations, but often it was not enough to handle the daily need.

For years, Maribelle's grandma stood behind a folding table and handed out her homemade dishes, which she cooked from each issue of *Southern Living* magazine. Everyone always managed to leave fat as a tick after enjoying her meals. And the last conversation she'd with Grams was that she wanted to follow in her footsteps. The only issue was, Maribelle, was not a chef like Grams, not by even the worst cooks' standards.

"You know what would be a big help with this goal?" Bridget offered, flipping through the glossy pages.

Maribelle didn't bother making eye contact. She knew the answer. "A man will not help."

"A man always helps." Bridget winked and used her thumb to touch the sparkling band on her finger. "It's alright; you don't have to believe me. Just wait, I'll prove you wrong."

"Yes, I'm sure when I'm eighty-three, you'll finally be right because by then I'll be too old to care about who I date." Maribelle stuck her tongue out. "Now, help me make a shopping list."

"Perfect!" Bridget grasped her hands together. "The best place to meet a man is at the grocery store."

Maribelle huffed and grabbed a pad of paper and pen from the kitchen junk drawer. As she closed the drawer, something caught her eye. A photo wedged up against the side. *Perfect timing*.

She removed the photo, her with Kurt and waved it at Bridget. "Photo evidence of my horrible luck with men and why starting off the New Year kissing a man is a terrible idea."

Bridget sprung from the couch and plucked the photo from Maribelle's hand. "This gorgeous couple is photo evidence of —"

Maribelle snatched the photo back. "Evidence of how much I've been heartbroken this year."

"You didn't know Kurt's dream of finding himself was by hiking through Africa. He completely pulled it from nowhere. However, he did want you to come with."

"The thought of hiking the Appalachian Mountains makes me short-winded. And it's not even hot out." Maribelle flipped open the trash can with her foot and tossed the photo inside. The lid slammed shut, another reminder of their relationship being over.

"Well, you won't get winded going to the New Year's Eve celebration on the Foley beach. You can handle that walk, right?" Bridget marveled.

Maribelle returned to the couch with her pad of paper and pen. "Count me out."

"No, not this year. I'll have you arrested and brought out there if I need to. I'll even make Shawn put on the lights and siren."

Ever since Bridget and Shawn started dating, she threatened to have people arrested.

"Brig, I don't want to celebrate New Year's Eve with a bunch of kissing couples." She put tomatoes, garlic, thyme, and oregano onto the list. "My tears will mix with the ocean water, and y'all will drown."

"Perfect, I'd love a midnight swim." Bridget leaned above the stack and hugged Maribelle, causing the magazines between to fall over. "I'm sorry, but seriously, you have to come. We've been talking about attending the celebration out there since we met, and I can't wait another year longer. We've celebrated New Years together since we became friends. It's a traditionI don't want to end. Plus, I bet there'll be single guys there."

"I'm not kissing a stranger." Maribelle placed her hand to her chest.

"After you kiss them, they won't be a stranger." Bridget took a magazine and leaned back into the couch pillows. "Relax, I'll make sure it's a cute stranger."

Maribelle rolled her eyes, continued to read recipes, and write down the ingredients. "Thank goodness I inherited Gram's bakeware. Otherwise, everything would've been cooked in either my mom's leftover Rubbermaid or to-go containers."

"You know the reason why you always have failing relationships, right?" Bridget asked, her eyes peeking over the magazine. "Because you can't cook."

"That's rather extreme. First, it's twenty-nineteen, women can do more than cook and keep house. Second, explain how any new relationship will not be the same as Jason and Kurt?"

"You couldn't have predicted Kurt's Africa journey. And Jason spent every minute of the day spreading his charm all around Charleston instead of being honest with you. He was far from ready for a relationship."

She wished it hadn't taken six months to figure out Jason's ways. It only made it harder to get over him. Plus, it left a scar of cheated worry across her heart for the next boyfriend. Maribelle wanted nothing to do with men, especially on New Year's Eve. She would go out single and start off single.

This New Year needed to begin better than last year. Although last year's New Year's Eve started out fun, hanging out with Bridget and friends. There must've been fifty people at her house, but everything turned south seconds before the midnight kiss. Maribelle had hoped that when Kurt took her hand in his, the words were going to be, will you marry me. Instead, Kurt stated he was leaving for Africa and asked her to go with him. He obviously thought she would jump at the chance to, but it only showed he didn't know her well at all. She could never leave Charleston, it was home.

"This week, I'm focusing on cooking and not worry one minute about a relationship." And she would continue to find a way to get out of spending it on the beach, even if it made her a horrible best friend.

"Don't worry about it at all. I'll find you the perfect guy." Bridget draped a blanket over her lap. "I mean, maybe that's been the issue all along, you haven't let me be your matchmaker."

Maribelle picked up a throw pillow with the word JOY embossed on it and chucked it at Bridget.

"Don't throw your joy at me." Bridget giggled as the pillow smacked her arm.

Maribelle laughed right along with Bridget as she tried to finish writing the grocery list. While Bridget made her feel like she was running out of time to find a man, Maribelle was running out of time to hit her New Year's goal.

Two

With her grocery list three pages long, Maribelle pulled a buggy from the stall, while Bridget grabbed one too. There was no way all the items she needed would fit into one. Hopefully, Maribelle's tiny eco-friendly car would hold all the groceries.

The store's Christmas decor was still up, but they added cases of champagne to the displays with large banners declaring Happy New Year. *Did they really need to remind people about the New Year? Who would forget?* The girls pushed the buggies up and down the aisles collecting ingredients from the list.

As they turned the corner to the next aisle, Bridget's hand grabbed Maribelle's elbow. "Look, he's cute."

Maribelle glanced up from her list and spotted the only other person in the pasta aisle. A man, about six-foot-tall, wearing jeans and an unzipped black hooded sweater. He stood in front of the sauce jars.

"Don't you dare," Maribelle whispered.

Bridget had zero qualms with approaching strangers and striking up conversations. Half of Maribelle's dates started this way. Any man was a target, from newborn to the elderly. Until she met Bridget, she'd no idea one could have a conversation with a baby.

Her best friend started to walk forward as Maribelle grabbed the back of Bridget's arm.

"No, no, no," Maribelle warned in a whisper.

Bridget shook Maribelle's hand free and continued down the aisle as though she was heading towards a groom at the altar. Maribelle spun toward the shelf and tried to hide her face with her list. What part of no did Bridget not understand?

"Hi, you should ask my single best friend, Maribelle, which sauce is best. She loves spaghetti." Bridget's voice traveled through the empty store.

Maribelle peeked around the list, watching for the stranger's reaction. The man glanced up at Bridget, and his eyes squinted as if questioning why this lady was approaching him.

Bridget pointed toward Maribelle, and she shoved the list back up over her face.

"I'm Davis." He leaned back around Bridget, making eye contact with Maribelle.

"I'm Bridget, and, of course, this is Maribelle," she waved, "Maribelle come say hi to Davis."

Maribelle grunted before pushing the buggy over. "Hi, I'm sorry for my friend here. She has a habit of running my life. Everyone's life."

"Do you have any plans for New Year's Eve?" Bridget asked, facing Davis.

"I declare!" Maribelle scolded. He could be married, but after peeking at his left hand, she didn't see a ring, or even a ring line tan, where one might have been.

Davis glanced between Maribelle and Bridget. "I don't have any plans. Do you have something in mind?"

Maribelle felt her cheeks warm, and she drew her attention back to her list. *How is Davis not put off by any of this?* So what if he was cute from afar and super cute up close. *Remember Jason and Kurt.*

"We're going to be a New Year's Eve celebration on the Foley beach." Bridget glanced over at Maribelle. She glared at Maribelle from the corner of her eye.

"I've always wanted to go to that, but usually I'm working," Davis cocked a smile.

"Then you must come. Maribelle needs a date."

72

Maribelle's eyes widen as she shook her head. "No, I don't need a date. I'll be recovering from my dish making excursion. Thank you for being so kind and entertaining Bridget. We need to finish shopping, so if you'd excuse us." Maribelle turned her cart the opposite way.

"Don't be rude," Bridget warned, causing Maribelle to pivot back around.

Davis moved closer to Maribelle, and it became more apparent how tall he was compared to her. Not to mention he smelled like rain in the woods, crisp and fresh. "Honestly, it would be nice if I could spend New Year's Eve on the beach. This is the first time I'm not scheduled to work."

Maribelle sighed and swallowed loud enough that she swore it echoed through the store. "It's definitely something to celebrate; having time off."

"How about I give you my phone number." He smiled. "If you decide you want to stand next to me on the beach, great, no strings attached."

Great, he's charming. "I can't say no if you want to stand on the beach." Maribelle lifted her shoulders in a shrug, trying to play it off as not a big deal.

Bridget snatched Maribelle's cell phone from her pocketbook before she could react. She entered Davis's name and number into the phone and handed it back to Maribelle.

"And in case you need to have me checked out, for safety's sake, my last name is Montgomery. The guy I paid to clear my name of all the arrests should have done so by now."

Maribelle juggled her phone, his joke catching her off guard. Bridget chuckled.

Davis shook his head. "I'm sorry, I'm horrible with jokes."

Bridget drew closer to them. "No worries, Davis. I'll have my fiancé run a background check."

Davis chuckled and returned to the shelf of sauce. "I'll let you ladies finish your shopping. You're buying enough food to feed half the town. But I hope to hear from you, Maribelle."

"You will." Bridget winked at her best friend. "I'll make sure of it. You two would make a cute couple."

"Again, I'm so sorry for the words that spill out of Bridget's mouth." Maribelle pushed the cart forward. "She thinks she runs the world."

"Not the world, just a few lives." Bridget beamed. "Now what is it that you do for a living, Davis?"

"I'm a chef." He placed a jar of sauce in his basket.

Maribelle choked on her saliva as Bridget patted her back.

"This is perfect," Bridget stated. "Maribelle is on a cooking and baking frenzy to complete her New Year's goal before the New Year. Talk about divine intervention. I bet Grams had something to do with this."

The thought of Grams being her guardian angel warmed Maribelle's heart. But it also made Maribelle realize she had to complete her goal before the New Year. She'd let her Grams down more times than she could count or wanted to remember. Maribelle never took the time to learn how to cook and bake. Even as a child, Grams would have her over, set everything up to teach her a recipe, and within minutes, Maribelle was bored and begging to play on the tree swing or with her dollhouse.

Maribelle couldn't recall a time when she showed interest in anything kitchen related and while Grams said it was not a big deal, she knew it was. It was the reason Grams left everything from her kitchen to Maribelle. If Maribelle couldn't make it a reality when her grandma was alive, she could at least do it one now, to honor her. And Maribelle couldn't put it off like everything else.

Bridget nearly yanked Maribelle's arm from her socket. "I bet he could help you out with your goal."

Maribelle waved her hands frantically. "Oh, no. We just met." *And he's already giving me butterflies in my stomach!*

"Perfect, what a great way to get to know each other before New Year's Eve, than by working in the kitchen together." Bridget beamed, looking over at Davis.

"I'm always able to help." Davis shifted the basket from his left hand to his right.

"Thank you, honestly, but we don't know each other, and I certainly can't invite a stranger over to my place. Let alone use you for your talents." Maribelle squeezed the buggy's handle until her knuckles were white.

Maribelle needed to focus on her goal. It was only six days then she could do whatever she wanted to do come the New Year. As Maribelle reached her hand up and attempted to run it through her hair, she remembered the messy bun piled on top. *Great first impression.*

"No pressure, you have my number if you change your mind. Have a great rest of your day, Maribelle and Bridget."

Davis took two steps backward and then pivoted around and headed out of the aisle. Maribelle caught him glancing back and making eye contact with her as he turned the corner.

"I can't believe you," Maribelle scolded.

"Yes, you can." Bridget leaned against her and wrapped her arm around her best friend. "That's why you love me."

It was true, so many great things came about in life thanks to her bold-talking best friend. Maribelle stopped pushing the buggy and pulled Bridget into a full hug. "You're an amazing best friend who always has my back, but you still drive me nuts."

Bridget winked and pushed her buggy forward, skipping behind it like a child.

Three

It took five minutes to lug all the groceries into her apartment, but it seemed like an hour.

Maribelle flopped on the couch and covered herself up with a peach-colored throw. She was far too tired from shopping to bother starting a recipe. At least Bridget had helped her load up the car.

"How do people shop *and* cook?" she asked aloud as she clicked the remote to the TV on. Maribelle settled on a Christmas movie re-run and pondered building a fire in the fireplace. She picked up her cell phone and checked the time when a text from Bridget popped up.

BRIDGET: I hope you've started cooking by now.

Maribelle sighed and sank further into the couch, trying to hide from her responsibilities, yet again.

Inside her refrigerator sat leftover take-out containers and meals her Mama had dropped off. Her freezer held packages of microwave dinners and ice cream sandwiches. Maribelle tried to think if she ran across a recipe that called for ice cream sandwiches.

MARIBELLE: Just about ready.

BRIDGET: Text Davis, I'm sure he'd love to help. He is soooo cute too.

Of course he's cute. Of course, I've thought of Davis every minute since we met. She envisioned them together in her kitchen going over recipes. She thought about how Davis might stand behind her and guide her hand as they stirred ingredients. Maybe even a fun little food fight filled with laughter. However, if Maribelle admitted that to Bridget she'd intervene even more. She didn't want a forced relationship. Maribelle wanted a relationship to form organically.

MARIBELLE: I'm not texting him, that's crazy.

BRIDGET: It would make your New Year's Eve date a lot better if you get to know each other a bit beforehand.

"New Year's Eve date-shmate!" she declared to the phone.

MARIBELLE: Don't you have some wedding planning to do?

BRIDGET: Don't you have some recipes to make?

Maribelle tossed her cell phone at a snowflake designed pillow and focused on the movie. She should've promised her Grams something that involved procrastination.

The thought of Davis twinkled in her mind like the Christmas lights around her fireplace mantel. She couldn't believe her luck of running into someone, not only handsome, but a chef. A part of her loved that Bridget had been with her and introduced them. The other part of her worried Davis would turn into something that would end like all the rest. She contemplated texting him.

Maybe if they went out to dinner, or some kind of date before New Year's Eve, she could get everything over and done. Start the year off correctly. Safely single. Yet, thanks to putting her goal off all year she was left with only six days. And she didn't have the time to do anything but complete her goal.

Maribelle picked up the December 1971 issue of *Southern Living* and thumbed to her marked spot. After reading through the recipes for a second time, she set off into the kitchen. As she set the Dutch oven on the stove, her cell rang.

She leaned over the back of the couch and noticed the screen read: Mama's Cell.

"Hi, Mama. How are you doing?" Maribelle returned to the kitchen and finally began unloading the groceries from the bags.

"I'm good, sweetheart. How are you?"

"Well," Maribelle opened the refrigerator door. "I'm finally starting on my promise to Grams."

"Sweetheart, that's great, but you know Grams loved you exactly as you are. You don't need to set your apartment ablaze to prove anything."

"Mama, I won't be setting anything on fire." *On purpose.*

"Do you want me to come over and help you?"

That was the last thing she wanted her mama to do. She loved her more than anything, but the second Mama stepped into the kitchen Maribelle might as well grab a cocktail and start a movie marathon. The opposite of completing her goal. Her mama could cook, taught by none other than Grams. Clearly, the homemaking apple fell off the family tree and rolled away when she was born.

"Thank you, Mama, but I need to do this on my own. No help."

"Alright, sweetheart, but if you change your mind, I'll be right over. Now, for New Year's Eve, are you planning on spending it with Bridget and her fiancé? Daddy wanted to make sure you knew you're invited over."

A whole chicken nearly slipped from Maribelle's free hand. She fumbled with it as the cell phone fell from her grasp and bounced across the kitchen floor.

"Sorry, Mama!" Maribelle hollered as she set the chicken safely into the refrigerator and picked her phone back up. She checked the screen—not a crack in sight—and let out a sigh of relief. The thick phone case had done its job. "Dropped my phone, I'm back. And no, you and Daddy hang out on New Year's Eve. I'm not sure of my plans yet."

"You can't spend New Year's Eve alone. You're always with Bridget. She and Shawn are welcome too."

A part of Maribelle was excited about spending the night of celebration alone. Thinking back, she'd never spent one alone. Plus, every New Year's Eve she'd spent with a man only lead to heartbreak shortly afterward. This year would be different; the only heartbreak she would experience would be a mouthful of horribly cooked food.

"Mama, I'll be fine. Now, I must go. These recipes won't cook themselves."

"Alright, sweetheart. Call if you need me."

I won't.

"Love you, Maribelle."

"Love you too, Mama. Bye."

Maribelle poured herself a glass of Merlot and leaned on the counter as she read through the recipe one final time. It felt like reading the airplane emergency card. She'd hate to miss something. The thought of Davis and his smile popped into her mind, causing her to reach for her phone. She tapped the internet icon and typed Davis Montgomery into the search bar. Maribelle bit her lower lip in anticipation.

Using her thumb, she clicked on the first link. As the page loaded, a juicy burger filled the screen along with the words: Montgomery's Place. She scanned the page. His place was located on Pine Street, a short ten-minute walk from her apartment. She was certain she'd passed it more times than she could count, but couldn't recall ever eating there.

Maribelle's eyes widened and mouth watered as she looked over the online menu. She and Bridget would need to stop by for a meal, unannounced of course. Davis's restaurant had to be fairly new as she continued to rack her brain, wondering why or how she'd never been there. She tapped on ABOUT and Davis's perfection appeared. He stood, both hands leaning forward on a counter, white chef's apron on. Behind him a stainless kitchen. As she stared into his eyes, Maribelle couldn't help but smile.

"Focus on your recipes," she snapped, set her phone down, and took a long sip of wine.

Maribelle pulled each ingredient she needed for the Chicken-and-Collards Pilau dish and lined it up on the counter. The directions seemed somewhat straight forward.

"Cook sausage in the Dutch oven, remove, and drain."

She plopped the meat in and turned the stove's burner to medium. Then she snatched her wine glass off the counter and waited. The recipe didn't say anything other than to cook it, and it's not possible to stir a sausage.

The sausage made a loud sizzle noise, and the apartment began to smell like never before; like home-cooked food. However, it quickly turned into the smell of something burning.

Maribelle lifted the lid off the Dutch oven to find a wrinkled up sausage at the bottom of chard bakeware.

"No, no, no!" Maribelle fanned the stove with her oven mitt and clicked off the burner. Re-reading the recipe, "Shoot, I missed the part about cutting up the sausage," she fanned the remaining smoke. "Your oxygen mask will now drop from the oven's hood."

Maribelle chucked the dish towel across the room and stomped her foot. "I'm sorry Grams," she said to the ceiling. "I fail at cooking. I fail at relationships. What's new?"

She glanced around at all of Grams's bakeware and stacks of *Southern Living* magazines. Why couldn't she be more like her and Mama? Grams managed to be a wife, cook, housekeeper, gardener, sewer, decorator, and mother. Maribelle managed to be a teacher, daughter, and dog mama to her dearly missed Maxwell. However, that had been the starting and stopping point.

She pulled at the middle of her sweater. Even Grams had fashion sense. All Maribelle had was comfy chic. Grams' nails were always done up in red polish, her lips in a rose peach color and her bleach blonde hair perfectly curled. Maribelle examined her nails. She kept them short to keep the classroom kids' dirt and glitter from getting underneath them. The fact that her toenails were painted was a Christmas miracle.

While Maribelle knew her Grams always loved her and was proud of her, there'd been moments when she knew her grandma expected more from her, even as a grandchild. The thing was, Maribelle wanted to be everything her Grams was, but the bar was set so incredibly high. All Maribelle could do was her best, and hoped that somewhere, somehow, Grams would approve.

Maybe the Handsome Chef had been her Grams providing a helping hand. Or at least some cooking tip helpers. As long as it didn't go any further than that. Ignoring the sausage mishap, and continuing with the recipe, she kept her phone nearby, just in case.

Four

She'd already deleted four texts to Davis as she sat at the kitchen island. The entire room smelled of burnt meat and disappointment. Maribelle topped off her glass of wine with Merlot. Crossing her arms, she gazed around at the mess of dishes and ingredients spread from the stove to the sink. A photo of Grams and her stuck to the refrigerator door caused her to type out the message to Davis once more, only this time, she hit send.

I'm only asking for guidance, and there's nothing wrong with that. Just a simple, can I call you for some advice on cooking?

Maribelle wasn't asking for a date or even inviting him over. She only wanted to figure out how to make the silly Chicken-and-Collards Pilau recipe.

Realizing he didn't have her number and won't know who the text was from, she quickly texted: It's Maribelle, from the grocery store a few hours ago.

DAVIS: Hi Maribelle, sure, please feel free to call me with any questions.

She felt all of the blood in her entire body rush directly to her face, and she fanned herself with a July 1988 issue. *Stop it, you're ridiculous. It's a call, not a proposal.*

Taking her phone, she thumbed over to the green phone icon and hit send.

He picked up on the first ring. "Hey, Maribelle." The perfect assertive, but nice voice danced in her ear.

"Hi, Davis, thanks, I know this seems weird, we just met, but I'm a lousy cook, and I took on this insane goal—" realizing her rambling, Maribelle cleared her throat. "I needed to know why my collard greens taste like bitter ocean seaweed. I followed the directions."

"How do you know what ocean seaweed tastes like?"

Maribelle laughed. "I'm just assuming it tastes similar to the horribleness I tempted to make."

"Try adding some extra salt or lemon juice," Davis suggested.

"Great, thanks. And the pilau I made with it tastes like a rubber sole." She stuck out her tongue and gave a silent blah.

"Maybe you should come over to my restaurant. I'm concerned that you're eating shoes and seaweed."

"Thank you for your concern." She wanted nothing more than to check out his restaurant, but no, she had too much to do and could already feel herself wanting to flirt with him. And flirting only led to heartbreak. "I promise I eat regular food."

"Good. Okay, for the pilau you can't remove the lid. It's super picky rice and any steam escaping messes up the two to one ratio of water and rice. Next time, stir it and then walk away."

"Thanks, that explains a lot." She took a sip of wine. "I'm sorry about Bridget earlier at the store. She can be a bit upfront about things. You don't have to join me for New Year's Eve."

"That's a shame. I'd already picked out my best party hat."

She giggled and covered her mouth. "I'm going to be so busy trying to get all these recipes done. Though, I feel bad about your hat going to waste."

A commotion of pots and shouting came through the phone, and Maribelle held it away from her ear.

"Sorry, I gotta go. Luke just dropped a tray of plates, and there's a mess everywhere."

Before she could say bye, Davis had hung up. Maribelle pouted with regret. She shouldn't have interrupted him during work. He was kind enough to answer, but whatever crashed in the background caused guilt to wrap around her. She should've figured it all out on her own. Maribelle needed to stick to the goal, cook the recipes. They didn't need to taste perfect. She wasn't Grams and the church would be grateful for the meals as long as they were edible.

Maribelle refocused. She straightened up the kitchen, washed the Dutch oven, and then moved onto the next recipe. She sent a prayer to Grams that this one would come out edible.

A knock at her apartment door startled Maribelle as she juggled a bag of flour in one hand and two sticks of butter in the other. She fumbled with the door handle and lock, popping it open with her foot. Staring right at her, was a puppy with golden eyes and a black and tan mixed muzzle.

"Love me!" Bridget's voice came from behind the mutt as she hoisted it toward Maribelle.

Balancing the butter on top of the bag of flour, she allowed Bridget to set the roughly ten-pound mutt into the crook of her arm. "What's this?"

"A puppy." Bridget reached for something on the other side of the door frame. "Two for one deal at the shelter." She held a tiny white ball of fluff in her arm.

Taking the mutt, flour, and butter with her, Maribelle walked to the kitchen. "No, Brig, you can't keep saving all these animals."

"I'm not saving allllll of them. Just two." Bridget leaned over the white dog and kissed its head.

"Just two this trip." Maribelle inspected the mutt in her head. Her heart ached at his cuteness.

Bridget's home contained three cats, four dogs, a parrot, and her fiancé. This white ball of fluff made dog number five.

"I can't have a dog." As if protesting, the mutt licked Maribelle's chin. "We discussed this."

"You can have a dog as long as it's less than thirty pounds. I double-checked with your landlord. No more making excuses. Plus I double-checked with your landlord." Bridget scrunched up her face. "What piece of furniture did you burn?"

Maribelle took the mutt with her and sat on the edge of her couch. "I tried to make Chicken-and-Collard Pilau, and it ended up more like Chicken-and-Seaweed Shoe."

"Oh, I heard that dish is all the rage this year." Bridget snickered. "Why didn't you call Handsome Chef?"

"I texted Handsome—Davis, and then I called him. He was kind enough to let me know what I did wrong."

"And?" Bridget crossed her legs and set the ball of fluff on her lap.

"And, he hung up on me. But I think I caused a distraction."

"Ouch." Bridget frowned, stroking the puppy's fur. "He didn't seem like that at the store."

"His restaurant sounded super busy, I shouldn't have bugged him. Anyways, it doesn't matter. I have to focus on my goal and now, apparently a puppy."

"Let's make a deal, so at least I get something for knowing my best friend isn't alone. Either accept the dog or spend New Year's Eve with Handsome Chef. Davis made a great first impression. Forget about the phone call. Imagine if you tried to handle a phone call in the middle of class. I'm letting you off easy."

Maribelle lifted the puppy; her hands cupped around its body and lowered it down with a kiss on his muzzle. "How about no to both? Come on, Brig you know I don't—"

"I know you don't what? You love dogs, and you've had such a rough year. This is way better than the perfume set and day spa certificate I gave you for Christmas anyway. Besides, once you finish your recipe goal, you'll have plenty of time for the puppy since you won't be dating. Although, I do approve of Handsome Chef."

Maribelle knew Bridget was correct. She did miss having a dog in her life. She glanced at the framed photo of her and Maxwell resting on the fireplace mantel. He'd been a rescue dog who lived a long and happy life until last spring. "Okay, I'll take this sweet guy."

"Yay! I knew it. Okay, I need to get ready for my one o'clock meeting."

Bridget, an interior designer, owned her own company. Which meant she could work any hours she wanted.

"While you're working on cooking ocean shoes, make sure you give that pup a proper name. We don't need a repeat of Maxwell."

"Maxwell enjoyed being nameless for a month. It gave him a purpose to strive hard to stand out."

Bridget raised an eyebrow as she slung her purse over her shoulder. She leaned in and hugged Maribelle goodbye. "Call me if you need anything. And light a candle or something, it smells horrid in here." Bridget waved and let herself out.

The door shut as Maribelle turned to the mutt resting in her lap. His fur was a colored mess of white and brown, like a well-mixed dish on the cover of *Southern Living*. She tilted her head. "What if I name you Pilau?" The pup opened his tired eyes and looked at her before resting his head back down. "Pilau it is, at least I can't mess this up." If only she could be as great in the kitchen as she was with a dog.

Five

M aribelle brushed the powdered sugar from her forehead with the back of her palm. She continued to mix, by hand, the frosting for the Coca-Cola cake she'd set on the counter to cool. Grams's stand mixer rested nearby, a ring of sugar in a crescent shape around it. It would take more time than she had to figure out how to work it without an eruption of sugar everywhere.

Pilau rested on the rug in the front of the kitchen sink. He'd not left her side since Bridget dropped him off yesterday afternoon.

"As soon as I get this mixed, we can head over to the little park across the street." Her apartment hosted a small patio area with some shade and gravel, but she wanted Pilau to be free to romp in some grass. Besides she needed to stretch her legs and breathe some non-burnt air.

After she frosted the cake, she stood back and examined her work. "It looks and smells edible." She smiled and placed the lid over the top of the container, locking it closed. "Alright, Pilau. We'll drop this at the church along with the cornbread and hush puppies, and then hit the park."

Maribelle took Maxwell's old leash from the coat closet and hooked it to Pilau's collar. She paused and took a deep breath. This would be the first time walking a dog since spring, and she fought back emotions of joy and sorrow. Bridget had been right; a dog was exactly what she needed, not a man. "If only you could cook, Pilau."

As they walked to the park, Pilau pulled the entire way, letting her know, this was his first time on a leash. The park couldn't have been more perfect, and a little rain would not keep her and the dog home. Besides with the rain she didn't need to worry about too many people around. She needed to learn Pilau's temperament with other people and animals, but based on the shelter information sheet, he did well being tested with kids, cats, and two dogs.

As they stepped off the sidewalk onto the grass, Maribelle un-clipped Pilau's leash. The park was fairly safe to keep a dog from running off. The trees made a natural fence of sorts with benches between each. But the way he stuck to her like glue, she didn't expect him to take off.

A well-weathered orange tennis ball smacked into her shoe, followed by a charging black Lab. "Hi, there big fella." She reached for Pilau, scooping him up before the Lab made contact.

"I'm so sorry. He's quite the fetch freak." A man approached. His eyes were covered by a baseball hat.

"Maribelle?" Davis squinted.

"Hey, funny seeing you here. Is this your dog?"

"Yes, this is Hank. Oh, you have a dog too. Don't worry; Hank is a sweet boy, no aggression."

Maribelle set Pilau on the grass and let the dogs sniff each other out. Both didn't show any signs of fear, and soon Hank flopped on his belly as if to say 'now we're the same height.'

"You remember Bridget. She has this thing about trying to save all the animals. But, I've only had him for a day and already love him. So I should say it's a blessing."

Davis smiled. "Hank's a rescue too." He shoved his hands in his pockets. "I wanted to apologize for the phone call yesterday. I didn't mean to hang up on you. When Luke dropped all the dishes, he cut his hand pretty bad and had to go to the emergency room."

"Oh gosh, is he alright?"

"Yes, all stitched up now. Thanks for asking. Anyways, sorry about hanging up on you."

"No, I'm sorry to have called you at work. You had plenty on your plate." She blushed.

"Nonsense, you needed my help. Maybe we can grab a bite to eat, work on some recipes before the New Year's Eve party. We can still go together, right?"

Her brow creased, now that she had Pilau, she worried about how he might be with fireworks, not to mention she'd be elbows deep in recipes up until the stroke of midnight. "It's not that I don't want to but—"

"But, you don't want to." Davis stared at the ground.

"No, it's not that." She touched his arm. "I have all these dishes to make, and honestly I'm the most boring person to hang out with in general, let alone on New Year's Eve. I mean, I don't even own a party hat like you."

Davis chuckled and rubbed the scruff on his chin. "You know my restaurant's closed on Mondays. If you wanted to bring your recipes over we could tag-team them and then enjoy a meal together."

Maribelle bit her lower lip.

"The goal you promised your grandma, didn't say anything about getting help, did it? I can be there for verbal guidance. I'll allow you to do all the work. If it makes you feel better, you can even bring your pots and pans."

"Two birds, one stone?" Maribelle glanced down at Pilau romping with Hank.

"A professional stone, with more ovens and burners than you could ever imagine." He winked, and she nearly fainted. *Handsome Chef alright.* "We can decide on New Year's Eve later."

Maribelle smiled. "Sounds great. Thank you. Speaking of recipes, I'd better get going."

"What did you name the new man in your life?"

Handsome Chef. "Pilau."

He grinned. "Oh that's clever, and it works well too. I'm glad you went with that over Collard."

She giggled. "Me too." Maribelle clipped on Pilau's leash and started to walk backward. "Great running into you and Hank." If she didn't leave immediately Maribelle knew she would start to either flirt or stumble over her words trying to keep her stomach butterflies at bay.

"The pleasure was definitely ours. See you tomorrow, Maribelle, about nine in the morning. You have the address."

"I do, thank you." She pivoted around and took all her strength not to skip her way back home. A warm smile formed on her lips and Maribelle pinched her eyes closed with excitement for her cooking lesson.

Six

M aribelle flipped the driver side mirror down and double-checked her make-up. She didn't put on too much,
but enough to make it look like she didn't just wake up and
drive right over to Davis's restaurant. The rain hit the car's
windshield in thick droplets as the palmetto trees danced the
tango in the wind. Jumping from the car, she made a mad dash
to the front door of Montgomery's Place.

The building sat two stories high. The front encased by
windows with lacquered black shutters. Oil lanterns were
unlit on either side of building's edge. She pounded her fist
on the door, assuming it would be locked. The rain continued
to dump from the gray sky.

The door swung open. "Come in." Davis moved aside.
"Goodness, it's nasty out there."

Maribelle stepped inside, but stood still, afraid to get water
all over the place.

"Let me take your jacket. Don't worry about getting anything wet. That's why it's tile flooring."

"Shoot, I left all the supplies in my car." She glanced over
her shoulder out the window.

Davis moved toward the door and pulled a long umbrella from a wooden holder. "How about you hold this and I'll grab everything."

As they stepped outside, Maribelle opened an umbrella big enough to be a circus tent. She popped the lock with her key and held the umbrella over his head and the bags as he carried them all in.

"That's it. Let's get you all set up." Davis took the umbrella from her and set it open to dry in the middle of the restaurant.

"This place is beautiful. I can't believe I haven't been in here."

The walls were white-washed brick. Deeply stained wood tables filled the middle with plush mismatched fabric chairs. From the ceiling, a mix of different size lanterns hung.

"It's only been open for about three months, so I won't fault you. But if it had been a year, then maybe." He winked.

Davis winked a lot, and she brought her hand to her cheek to hide the blushing it caused. If only she could keep her face from showing how adorable he looked when he winked. If there was something between her and Handsome Chef, she didn't want to go down that path, especially when she'd no doubt see him at the park and grocery store. They could be friends, though, the safest bet for her heart.

"Where's Pilau?"

"With my parents. I wasn't sure how he would do with the weather and didn't want to leave him all alone. How does Hank do with the storms?"

They moved past the tables and through the swinging door leading to the kitchen.

"He does excellent; his hearing is mostly gone so he can't hear the wind or thunder. I suppose he can feel it, but as long as he has his crate, he's good. He was the easiest dog ever to crate train. Some nights I find him in there instead of on the bed with me."

"I've never heard of a dog who likes a crate. Pilau doesn't have one. I should probably get him one soon. Once I'm back at work, he'll be home alone all day."

"What do you do?" Davis pulled two coffee mugs from the dish area.

"I'm a teacher over at Hilton Elementary."

"My mom's a teacher too, over in Columbia. She loves it." He poured black coffee into the mugs. "My dad thinks she should've retired years ago, but she figured why quit something you love just because of your age."

"Excellent point, but I'm looking forward to retirement, already." She accepted the mug from Davis.

"Cream? Sugar?"

"No, thanks. If it's not a latte, I like it straight." Maribelle lifted the mug in a cheer of sorts.

Davis copied. "I think we both have a ways to go before we can retire."

"Don't get me wrong, I love teaching, but I know by the time retirement age comes I'll be more than happy to hang up my teacher's cape."

Davis nodded and smiled. "Teacher's cape, I like it."

"I appreciate your help with this goal of mine. I've picked what I thought will be the hardest recipes from the magazines since I'm here with you."

Davis held his coffee mug and leaned back against a cook station. "I'm here to help if you need me."

"I want to do as much as possible on my own. Sounds rude, I know. You can give me all the instructions you see fit." Maribelle sipped the coffee, the rich flavor perfect on her taste buds.

"Are you the head chef of the kitchen now?"

"Maybe." This time Maribelle was the one giving a wink. "Alright. Chocolate lasagna recipe." She opened up *Southern Living* to the page and set it on the counter.

"That's an easy recipe."

"Says the chef." Maribelle's shoulders slumped. "Even spelling lasagna is hard." She read over the recipe. Sure it seemed simple, but anything involving cookie crumbs could be a mess. Davis stepped up behind her, and she could hear him breathing.

"Can I at least gather supplies for you?" His voice drifted over Maribelle's shoulder as his breath tickled her ear.

His nearness caused her stomach to tighten with anticipation.

Without turning around, "Yes please," she said.

He was causing her to lose focus quickly. She removed the ingredients from the bags and lined them up while Davis set a long glass dish and mixing bowls in front of her. The recipe called for crumbled chocolate sandwich cookies.

"Is there a specific way to crumble a cookie? And what about the creamy middle? Do we scrape it out?" She pointed at the recipe.

"Am I supposed to tell you?"

Maribelle glanced over her shoulder. "It would be helpful."

Davis stepped next to her, and their long sleeve shirts touched.

"You don't need to remove the filling, which would take forever, although it's my favorite part of the cookie."

"Mine too." She turned toward him. "I used to scrape out the middle with my teeth and throw the rest of the cookie away."

"Oh, that's wasteful." Davis's lips pouted.

Maribelle shook her head and turned back around. "I know."

"I used to take a butter knife, scrape out the middle, and make a creamy sandwich. Then with the cookies, I'd break them up and add them to a tall glass of milk."

She could picture a young Davis with a spoon, stirring up the mixture. Maribelle licked her lips, thinking about how good that must have tasted. She felt horrible for all those cookies she tossed. "Sounds like you have always been a chef."

Davis pointed toward the food processor, and she dumped the cookies into it. "I have, looking back on it. But I didn't know for sure until college."

Maribelle tilted her head, leaning in toward the food processor. "Do I want to use the low button?"

"I'd recommend pulse. It'll give you a better idea of when you're at the consistency you want."

She brought her finger to her chin. "I don't think the recipe says."

Davis grabbed a stool from a nearby workstation and sat down to her left. "You'll want it to between beach sand and rocks."

"Pebbles?"

Davis nodded and chuckled. "I'm guessing you eat a lot of takeout food."

"No." Maribelle huffed as she pushed the pulse button. "I microwave too."

Next, she grabbed the cream cheese, sugar, and whipped topping, and Davis pointed at a mixing bowl.

"Don't you have one of those fancy stand mixers? Grams left me her's. I didn't bring it because I figured you had one, and it's about twenty pounds. Plus, every time I use it, I make a mess. I'd hoped you could show me what I'm doing wrong."

"I have an industrial size one, but you need a small one for this." He handed her a hand mixer with two beaters. "And what you need to do with yours at home is start it at the slowest speed and cover it, or find the guard attachment."

She dropped the ingredients in the bowl and began to mix. The cream cheese instantly became stuck in the beater and threatened to twirl the bowl across the counter. As Maribelle reached for the bowl, Davis did too. His hand moved over top of her's. The butterflies inside her fluttered and sent chills down to her fingertips. Instead of switching the mixer button to a slower speed, she ramped it up to high. Even with both of their hands on the bowl, it tried to dance away. Maribelle switched the mixer to off as they started to laugh. The bowl waddled to a stop on the counter.

"Oh, goodness. I was not expecting that." Her hand still on the bowl.

"Me either. That takes talent." Davis raised an eyebrow at the bowl and turned to her.

Even his grin made her knees weak. She couldn't help but stare at him like a just-lit Christmas tree. But if she wanted to hit her goal, she could not get side-tracked. And she needed to not fall mixer-over-bowl for him.

She returned to the magazine and followed the instructions for hand mixing the butter with the cookie crumble. Next, she folded it into the pan. Then, Maribelle took a spatula and started to push the filling around on top of the crumble mixture. Yet, when she went to smooth it out, the crumble stuck to the crust, pulling it up into a messy wrap.

"Oh, no! That's not like the picture." She buried her face into her hand. "What can I do?"

Davis stood close enough for Maribelle to pick up a rustic evergreen wood scent. She closed her eyes for half a second and pictured them off hiking around, sharing a picnic lunch.

"Let's have you pipe it in. I never use a spatula."

"Well, we can't let this go to waste." She took the spatula full of cookie crumbles and cream cheese mixture, wiped some off, and licked her finger. Maribelle turned the spatula around and extended her arm toward him.

"That's a lot of sugar at once." Davis took his finger and wiped off a bit for himself.

She smiled as she wiped off more from her side of the spatula. "Yep, but worth it."

Davis chuckled and removed a clear, pointed bag with a metal tip from nearby and handed it over to Maribelle. "Filler-up."

She removed a long metal spoon from the rack on the counter and scooped the mixture into the plastic sleeve. "This is much easier. I already know without even spreading it yet."

"Make sure you—"

Maribelle held up her hand. "No, this I got." She rolled the top of the bag over twice and tilted her chin to the ceiling with pride. Maribelle squeezed the cream cheese mixture into the pan. With both of her hands now near the tip of the bag, the top unrolled and a large glob of it popped out and landed with a smack on her black ballerina flats. "No!"

"I hope you don't plan on licking that up too." Davis glanced at the mess below.

"Funny." She tapped his arm with the back of her hand.

"Try twisting the top closed. Rolling it doesn't work well, as you see."

Maribelle pointed her finger. "Excellent pro-tip. Thank you." She smirked and twisted the top of the bag closed and piped out the mixture onto the crumble topping.

Davis disappeared behind the storage of pots and pans, returning with several small white towels and wiped her shoe as clean as possible.

"Thank you; I've never had a gentleman clean my shoes before." She tucked her hair behind her ear.

"When this restaurant opened up, I think I ended up replacing about six pairs of tennis shoes while I tested and perfected recipes and trained staff. Everyone starts someplace."

"And everyone fails someplace else." Maribelle set the frosting bag on the counter.

A pounding from out in the dining room alerted them.

She waved him off as she turned to the lasagna dish. "I'll stay here and finish this or I'll never meet my goal." The kitchen door swung back and forth after Davis exited through it.

Who would be banging on the door in the middle of a storm. Maybe someone was stranded and needed help. Maybe a tree fell on someone's car. Or maybe ... maybe it was a girlfriend. *It couldn't be a girlfriend because he wants to go to the New Year's Eve party with me.* Davis seemed like the perfect man, helpful, funny, dog-friendly, chef, and handsome. *But he has to have at least a few women admirers.*

The chocolate lasagna called for instant pudding, and she made it, mixing it with great frustration. Maribelle not only realized that the recipe was rather easy, but that she was completely inept at making even the simplest recipes. Feeling her forehead wrinkle as she continued to scold herself, Maribelle dumped the pudding on top of the cream mixture.

"Maribelle." Davis entered the kitchen.

She swung around, facing him with the bowl in her hand. There she was, clearly, the girlfriend.

The mixture ran down the sides, onto her fingers and started to slip. Maribelle fumbled with the bowl as tossed it toward the edge of the counter with a clatter. Maribelle winced and looked over at them. And one who probably could cook. How'd she let herself entertain a hike and picnic in her mind? She knew better. She'd even told herself no relationships before the New Year. Why'd he agreed to come out with her on New Year's Eve if he had a girlfriend?

"Maribelle, this is Chelsea." Davis stood next to her, his arms at his side instead of around Chelsea's waist or shoulder. *Maybe they had a fight and that's why he didn't mention her.*

She hoped Davis would add the words: my sister. The kitchen remained as silent as rising bread.

"Chelsea, this is Maribelle. I'm helping her with her New Year's goal."

Chelsea shook Maribelle's hand. It was velvety soft as though she soaked it in milk all day. "Nice to meet you. I didn't mean to interrupt. Crazy storm outside and I noticed Davis's truck out front. My car's out of gas. I'd insert a blonde joke here, but I'm not a natural."

Maribelle stood still, her eyes focused on Chelesa's roots for her natural hair color.

"I'm going to take her over to pick up some gas. Are you alright if I leave you here to cook? You won't burn my restaurant down, will you?"

He's leaving me here, all alone, in his restaurant? "Are you sure, I mean I can go back home and cook. You barely know me well enough to leave me here."

"The storm is pretty bad; it's not safe out there." Concern spread across Davis's face. "Please stay, I'll be back in two shakes of a lamb."

"Tail," Chelsea added. "Lamb's tail."

"Tail?" Davis questioned. "I thought it was just two shakes of a lamb. You know when you season it and shake it off. You always give it two shakes."

Chelsea threw her head back laughing and then wrapped her arm around Davis's waist. "All these years and you still surprise me."

Before Maribelle could reply, Chelsea and Davis were out the kitchen's swinging door. And Maribelle couldn't move fast enough. *All these years?* She piled her remaining ingredients back into her bags, and then she finished the chocolate lasagna and snapped a lid onto the dish. She'd decided not to buy throw-away containers for her cooking and baking goal. With each donation to the church meal program, they could re-use her Grams dishes far better use than collecting dust in her kitchen.

By the time Maribelle had loaded up her car, she was sopping wet. Without Davis holding the umbrella the rain-soaked through every inch of fabric. Her ballet flats were clean of the whipped topping for sure. She took a deep breath and started the car. Chelesa might not be a girlfriend, but she was important to Davis and Maribelle would not be getting in the middle of it. Before she could back out of the spot, she paused, leaving the restaurant unlocked was not a good idea. Even if he'd clearly forgot to mention his girlfriend, she wasn't low enough to cause his business to be robbed or trashed. She decided to wait in her car until he came back.

Within a few minutes, a navy blue truck pulled up, and Davis climbed out. He dashed inside without even noticing Maribelle sitting in the car. She put the car in reverse. While the plan had been to drop off all the food at the church, she didn't want to embarrass herself by only offering up a tiny dessert. Instead, Maribelle headed straight to her parent's to pick up Pilau. She leaned over the steering wheel to try and see through the sheets of rain.

Once she changed clothing and placed the chocolate lasagna in the fridge, she turned off her cell phone in an attempt to shut out the world. She pulled a pint of Rocky Road from the freezer. It didn't matter how cold it was outside, or how many recipes she needed to make. For now, Maribelle was putting on a Hallmark movie and forgetting about everything in her life. Pilau curled up next to her on the couch.

"Maybe this goal, this promise to Grams was an impossible task. I can't be someone I'm not, I can't be Grams." She rubbed his back with one hand and shoveled ice cream into her mouth with the other. Maribelle counted how many remaining recipes she had and how many days were left. "I don't think this is possible, Pilau."

Seven

A pounding at Maribelle's door woke her up. On the coffee table rested an empty pint of ice cream with a spoon inside. Pilau let out a single puppy bark and dashed to the door with all ten pounds of fury. The pounding came again, and she threw off the blanket and went to the front door.

"I was worried about you." Bridget shoved her way inside, hugging her best friend before petting Pilau. "I knew you were out today, not only in this mess, but with Davis."

Maribelle rubbed her sleepy eyes awake and closed the door. "I'm sorry. I turned off my phone when I got home from picking up Pilau and accidentally fell asleep."

"Why did you turn off your phone in the middle of a storm?" Bridget removed her coat and hung it over the back of a chair and made her way to the couch.

"Handsome Chef has a girlfriend. Don't give me some lame excuse to try and explain it." The time on the microwave clock read one-thirty. She prepared the coffee and hit the switch. Maribelle waved an empty mug at Bridget.

"No thanks, it's way too late in the day for me." Bridget perched herself on the edge of the couch. "How do you know it's his girlfriend? After all, he did say he would go out with you on New Year's Eve."

"After she showed up, he left me alone in his restaurant."

"Who showed up?" Bridget picked up Pilau and cuddled with him on her lap.

"Chelsea. She ran out of gas." Maribelle added some peppermint coffee creamer to her mug.

"Does she not look at her dashboard?"

"I guess not." Maribelle poured more creamer into her mug. "So, I took off right after he left." She stuck a spoon in the mug and stirred. "Davis and I had this connection; I could feel it. Ughhh, I'm so stupid."

"How are you stupid? You know the rule. If you call yourself stupid, you need to explain why."

Maribelle plopped back onto the couch, leaned back, and crossed her arms. "You should've been a therapist, not an interior designer."

"Technically, I work with couches," Bridget smirked. "You're not stupid because you like a guy."

"I am when I specifically shouldn't have entertained the idea of Davis's help. Speaking of, I need to be cooking right now."

"Let's turn on your phone." Bridget swiped the cell phone off the coffee table and waved it in the air. "Davis has probably been trying to reach you if he came back to his restaurant and you were gone without warning. "

Maribelle snatched her cell from Bridget's grip. "No, it stays off. I've got to get to these recipes done, and I don't need any more distractions."

"What can I do to help?" Bridget glanced around. "Hold the fire extinguisher?"

"Not all of us are chef material." Maribelle sipped her coffee and opened up the *Southern Living* magazine to her next recipe. "Cooking and baking is a learned skill, which I'm still learning."

Bridget's cell beeped, and she slid it from her pocket. "Remember this is Charleston, I think home cooking is a mandatory skill for ladies."

"Grams sure made it seem that way." Maribelle grabbed a whole chicken from the refrigerator and set it on the counter.

Bridget nodded her head as she read the text on her phone. "Shoot, I've got a client asking me about swatches."

Maribelle glanced out the kitchen window as rain melted down the glass.

Bridget hugged Maribelle. "Turn your phone back on." She threaded on her coat over by the front door.

"I will in a few hours. You should be home safe by then, right?"

"Yes." Bridget stood, and Pilau waddled over to the door with her. "You know, it sucks that I'm losing you on New Year's Eve to Pilau, but I guess I understand."

"Do you?"

Bridget shook her head. "Nope." She kissed her hand and blew the air-kiss across the room. "Bye."

Before Maribelle could respond, Bridget was out the front door and down the hall. Pilau returned to the living room with what sounded like a bored sigh as he flopped down on the rug. "Sorry, you're lonely, bubba."

Maxwell came to mind as his photo caught her eye. She went to the hall closet and pulled out an unmarked box in the back. "You might like these, Pilau. A very special dog had them before you, and I know he would love you to have them." Squatting to the floor she turned the box upside down as a myriad of dog toys tumbled out.

"You entertain yourself while I start on Chicken n' Dumplings." She snatched the magazine off the couch. "I'm looking forward to this one."

She reviewed the recipe, which seemed easy, even for her. Maribelle filled the Dutch oven with water and set the bird inside. While it cooked, she started on the next recipe, Poppy Seed Chicken.

The rain didn't let up, and she turned her cell back on before lifting the boiled chicken from the Dutch oven. Her cell alerted her like a fire alarm as the text messages came in and voice mail beeped. Hesitant, she checked and found they were all from Davis. Her heart sank. Even if Chelsea was his girlfriend, she shouldn't have left him without a word. It was ugly of her to do and she knew it.

Maribelle returned to the couch, finished her coffee, and watched as Pilau had a blast with the toys. When the timer beeped, she removed the casserole dish from the oven. Maribelle removed the buttermilk biscuits from the refrigerator and popped the roll on the edge of the counter. Pilau let out a puppy size bark and jumped up.

"Sorry, bubba." The fact that she was no longer alone in the silence of her thoughts made her smile. Having Pilau had been what she needed all along. Maribelle laughed at the thought, as contented happiness spread through her.

After she shredded the whole chicken and added it back to the Dutch oven, she dropped the strips of cut up biscuit dough into the boiling chicken stock and covered it with the lid. Maribelle took a deep breath; the scent of home cooking instantly transported her back to times with Grams. Closing her eyes, she continued to take knowing breathes, allowing the smell to fill her nose. Her kitchen usually smelled like wet socks and soy sauce when she reheated her take-out leftovers.

As the biscuits cooked, Maribelle picked up her cell. Davis had texted her three times and left one voicemail. She deleted the voicemail without listening to it and did the same with the text messages. Reading or listening to him wouldn't change the way she felt or Chelsea's status. He was like every other man she dated, not a good match for one reason or another. "At least this year I can ring in the New Year with you." She stroked the puppy's fur; her fingers lost below it.

Pilau jumped off the couch and ran to the front door.

"Oh no, you must have to go potty." She dashed to the oven and turned off the burner and then threaded on her rain jacket. Since the back patio was a swamp, she'd have to take Pilau to the park. With her rain boots on, and umbrella in hand, the puppy and Maribelle made their way to the park.

The rain continued to come down in giant drops as she wrestled with keeping Davis out of her mind. Thinking back on them in the restaurant made her feel foolish. She'd read more into him offering to help her out than he did. *Maybe I should text him back. Give him the benefit of the doubt that I'd been the one that read the signals all wrong.*

"Maribelle."

She recognized the voice. It belonged to Davis.

Eight

A dripping wet Hank appeared in front of her and Pilau. He dropped his ball and shook the rain from his fur. Davis walked up and faced Maribelle.

"Why haven't you answered my texts? I was worried about you." Even while standing under the protection of the umbrella, the wind blew rain against Davis's jeans and jacket.

"How long have y'all been out here?" Maribelle questioned. "You're sopping wet."

"I didn't know where you lived, and you couldn't bother to return my text or calls, so I figured at some point Pilau, and you would have to take a potty walk, even in the storm."

The wind whistled, and both of their umbrellas attempted to turn inside out. Rain smacked Maribelle's cheeks and hair. She shivered as Pilau located a spot to use the restroom.

"Look, I'm sorry, Davis." She switched hands with the umbrella so she could see his face better. "I didn't leave your restaurant unattended. I waited in the car until you pulled up and ran inside. Then I left."

"But why did you leave?" He chucked the ball for Hank, who took off after it. "I was only gone a few minutes, and I needed to help Chelsea. She's a friend."

"A friend?"

"Dare I say a best friend? Her brother and I have been best friends since kindergarten, and she was kind of a package deal since they're twins."

"I thought she was your... a close friend. Maybe something more." Maribelle wanted to smack herself upside her own head.

Davis started to chuckle. "She's a sister to me, just like her brother, Clint. Chelsea is an awesome woman, but she and I would never date. We're complete opposites."

As the rain continued to soak them, Hank returned with his ball, dropping it at Davis's boots.

"I feel so silly for overreacting. It's just been a—"

"I wouldn't have asked you to get together for dinner or entertained the idea of the New Year's Eve party if I had a—" He chucked the ball again. "Close friend."

The wind hollowed and swept Maribelle's hair across her face.

"I'm sorry you had guys in your life that played games with your heart. Had I known, I would've introduced you to her as," he held his hand out like Vanna White, "Chelsea, not my girlfriend or anything romantic."

She glanced back at her apartment. "I just made Chicken n' Dumplings and I'd like to make up my stupid embarrassment by offering you dinner." While she'd planned to deliver it to the church, this certainly seemed like a viable excuse to keep a few bowls.

"Since it's my favorite dish, I must accept. But I don't have a change of clothes on me, and Hank is three times as much a mess as Pilau."

"A little water never hurt anyone, especially a southerner." She glanced down at the two mud-covered dogs. "They might be a different story."

As they made their way to her apartment, Pilau and Hank strolled at their owners' side. With the downpour and wind, their umbrellas were useless.

"This might be more than a little water," Davis said, standing inside the front door. "Gosh, it smells great in here."

Maribelle took Davis's jacket. "Thank you. I can honestly say no one has ever said that before here, even when I ordered in."

"Standing in the rain was beyond worth it."

"Don't judge too fast." She covered her mouth to hide a laugh. "It might smell good, but I'm not sure it's edible. I did follow the recipe exactly."

Hank and Pilau did a group shake, sending sprays of rain-soaked fur all over the place. She hurried off to the hall closet and pulled a stack of towels out and handed three to Davis and kept one to dry off Pilau. After he dried off Hank and she dried off Pilau, she shivered as her clothing was soaked through too. Thinking back, she couldn't recall such a stormy December. "I have some bigger clothes that should fit you if you don't mind."

Davis shrugged, and she couldn't make out if he was put off or not by it. She gathered a pair of super baggy sweats and an oversized t-shirt from the bottom drawer of her dresser. The shirt was lilac, but at least the sweats were an ashy gray.

"Should I ask why you have these?" Davis questioned taking them from her.

"No, probably not." She winked. "The bathroom is down the hall."

Maribelle didn't want anyone other than Bridget to know about her comfy clothing. The ones she wore when she didn't care about being southern chic and lady-like. Clothes she could eat all the ice cream, bacon, and mac and cheese in and not have to unbutton her pants or hold in her stomach. The clothes that were a few sizes too big. No, that secret would stay safe.

She hurried off into her bedroom to change from her wet clothes. When Maribelle returned to the living room, she found Hank and Pilau snuggled up on the rug together near the stack of toys. The aroma of Chicken n' Dumplings didn't even stir them awake, proving it was a long day for all.

"I believe the height difference between us is now incredibly noticeable."

Maribelle spun around to find Davis walking down the hall, the sweats so far from his ankles it appeared as though he was wearing super short jogger sweats.

"At least the shirt fits." She tried not to laugh.

"Not everywhere." He glanced at his shoulders, which looked like they were trying their darndest to not bust through the material. "Thankfully, dinner won't go straight to my shoulders."

Maribelle placed a hand on her hip. "Mine sure will. I see a ton of overweight shoulders."

Davis entered the living room with a chuckle.

"Would you like something to drink?" She moved into the kitchen and lifted the lid off the Dutch oven. Steam wafted up with the deliciousness scent of chicken and biscuits. "I think it's ready."

Davis approached and observed the Chicken n' Dumplings. "Oh, yes, it's perfect. Do you have any white wine? It would complement this meal nicely."

Maribelle opened the cupboard and removed two wine glasses. "I have a Chardonnay chilling in the fridge. If there is one thing I know, it's pairing wine with take-out food."

"Maybe you're a chef, after all. It's just been hidden. Wine pairings can be tricky." He leaned against the counter.

Maribelle blushed as she opened the wine bottle. "Actually, it's not a talent. It's called Pinterest. There are about a thousand boards on the subject."

"Fake it until you make it, right?" Davis took the glass half full of Chardonnay and examined the kitchen.

"I know it's a mess." Grams' bakeware was stacked here and there on the counter and the island between towers of *Southern Living* magazines. "But I'm only keeping a few of her dishes and donating the rest to the church filled with food."

"How wonderful, I love how much they help out the community with their daily free lunches."

"Do you ever have any leftovers you donate from your restaurant?"

"Sometimes." He sipped his wine. "It's still a work in progress to learn how much food I need to order to prevent waste. There's a steady flow into the restaurant lately. When I first opened, I donated many lunches to the church because I was learning what people wanted to eat and what they didn't. I've gotten better at judging amounts, but I continue to make a few trips to the church with donations."

She placed two bowls on the counter and scooped the chicken n' dumplings equally into each with a ladle. "I admire your ability to run a restaurant. I'm pretty sure I would fail before I even started."

Maribelle handed Davis his bowl. "Do you eat yours with a fork or spoon?"

"Spoon. Wait do you know people who eat it with a fork?" He tilted his head, taking the spoon from her hand.

"My Grams always served it with a spoon, but I've been to a few restaurants that served it with a fork in the bowl."

They headed into the dining room between the front door and the living room. The Christmas tree lights gave off a soft romantic glow around the apartment. Davis pulled out a chair at Maribelle's tiny wooden table and motioned for her to sit.

"Thank you, kind sir." She curtsied.

He bowed and pulled out his chair, sitting across from her. When she glanced up at him, he smiled shyly, and it made her blush. Maribelle took a long sip of wine to try and wait for her cheeks to cool off, but the alcohol only made them rosier.

"This is good," Davis stated, taking another bite of chicken n' dumplings.

"It is, right? Who would've thought." Maribelle blew on her spoonful.

"I did." He winked.

"Thank you. I'm starting to have fun making these recipes." She gazed off at the dogs sleeping. Nothing made her feel more at peace than sleeping pets.

"I love cooking, for a full restaurant, or a date."

"Do you cook for lots of dates?" Maribelle ran a hand through her damp hair. A slight curl had developed from the added moisture of being outside.

"No, dates are rare for me. Chelsea is always trying to set me up with someone. They're nice women, but no connections."

A part of Maribelle wished that was her issue instead of the disappear-ers and cheaters.

The Christmas tree lights caught the gleam in Davis's eyes. "Tell me what you like to do for fun? Blow off steam after all those kids."

"I love to golf. I think it's a rite of passage as a Charleston-ian."

Davis nodded in agreement. "Yes, it is, but I hate golf."

She laughed. "You do?"

"Shhh, don't tell my mama."

"If you don't golf, what do you do in your free time?" Maribelle leaned back in her chair, taking the wine glass in her hand.

"I read, a lot. I love to fish and work in my woodshop."

"You have a woodshop?"

"Yes. I make furniture in my spare time. Every man needs a few hobbies." He rested his elbow on the table.

"That sounds like a second career, not a hobby. I'm super impressed. Now whatever I say is going to be rather lame."

"I bet you have some great hobbies."

"I love to read also. And I told you about the golf. But I'm kind of a couch potato too. Bring me some food and wine, and I can chill all weekend without feeling guilty at all."

"Sounds like a fun date, if I'm not being too forward."

Maribelle didn't care if he was being forward or not, as she became lost in his eyes. Davis wasn't model perfect, he was man perfect. "What do you usually do on a date?"

He took a bite of dinner, and while she waited, Maribelle pondered what he would answer. Davis mentioned he cooked for his dates. Probably followed up by a movie out, or walk in the harbor.

"As you know, I cook for my dates, but usually that's as far as it goes. If I can't carry on a conversation for several hours over food and drinks, then for me, it won't work."

Maribelle couldn't recall a time when she and any date stayed and chatted over a long meal. Usually, the guy rushed her off to the movies or even a friend's party; which always felt uncomfortable since she didn't know anyone there.

"What about you?" He folded his hands over his bowl, the spoon hung between it.

"I enjoy a great meal, but I've never dated a man who cooked for me. We always went out. I love conversations. And I do like to go for strolls around the neighborhood." She covered her mouth with her hand, embarrassed. "I sound like I'm fifty-five."

"Not at all. I love neighborhood walks. I get a chance to say hi to my neighbors, and so does Hank. He loves attention."

"He's a sweet dog. I love that he and Pilau get along." This may not be a date, but she wanted it to be. Maribelle wanted to go on walks with Davis and Hank. She wanted to kiss Davis in the park and hold his hand under the stars.

"Maybe we all can be friends."

Friends? Well then, that answers that question. This is exactly why I told Bridget no New Year's Eve date. "I'm going to get some more wine. Can I get you any?" She forced her chair backward, bumping the wall behind it.

"Sure, thank you." Davis lifted his glass for her.

Maribelle flung open the refrigerator, pulled out the bottle, and topped off both of their glasses. She needed to not over-react. After all, they weren't dating and friends or not, New Year's Eve was no longer anything to even entertain. Thanks to Pilau saving her she could avoid it all together.

She handed him his glass and crashed back into her chair. "I have a lot of recipes left to cook before midnight on New Year's Eve."

"Anything I can help with? I'd be happy too." He immediately took a long sip of wine.

"Thanks, but I think I'm handling it rather well. And I'm sure you have wood to whittle or something." Her tone had changed, and she knew it. She shoved a bite of food into her mouth and stared at the sleeping dogs.

"Did I say something wrong?"

The enjoyable atmosphere continued to cave in around her. "No, it's been a long day," she snapped. *It has nothing to do with the fact that you only want to be friends.* "I'm sorry for being rude."

"We appreciate the warm home and dry clothes. Dinner was excellent. Please stop by my restaurant soon, and I'll make you something."

"Thank you."

He scooted his chair out and took his empty dishes to the kitchen and set them in the sink while she remained at the table. "I think it's best if Hank and I go." Davis patted his leg. Hank yawned and stretched as he stood up. Pilau lifted his head as if to ask, 'why is my friend leaving?'

Maribelle stood, and before she could react, Davis gave her a quick half-hug, grabbed his wet coat, and gave a half-wave goodbye. The door shut and she and Pilau started at it for what felt like minutes before Maribelle gained her composure.

"He left in my lounge clothes."

Nine

Maribelle spent the next several days baking and cooking like a hurricane. She battered the kitchen and kept the winds strong for about seventeen to eighteen hours, knocking out as many recipes as possible. Lord willing and the creek don't rise, was her motto.

And she only had eight recipes left to complete. Macaroni Pie, Chicken Fried Steak, Peanut Brittle, Quiche Lorraine, and Pineapple Casserole, to name a few. Anything to keep her mind from wandering to Davis.

She only left the apartment to drop off the dishes at the church and take Pilau to the park. The car's back seats were stacked high with dishes, taking a few trips to unload them all. On the drive back she couldn't help but glance over at Montgomery's Place, and spotted his truck parked out front. Luckily, she'd avoided seeing Hank and Davis at the park during their quick game of fetch.

Once back home, Maribelle clicked on the television for background noise as she looked around her apartment, the Christmas decorations still up.

"For someone who bases relationships on communication during the first date, you'd think he'd be better at it than he is." She knelt down and scratched Pilau's chin with both hands, his hind leg kicking with delight.

To say she grew to love cooking sounded odd, Maribelle had only been doing it for six days. But, Grams's spirit was surely around her, helping her, guiding her, somehow.

A knock at the door broke through her thoughts. "Come in," she called out, knowing it was Bridget who'd texted twenty minutes ago that she was on her way.

"Happy New Year's Eve Eve," Bridget said, entering. "I don't know why I brought over sandwiches for dinner. You've probably been snacking on recipes all day."

"Shouldn't you be in the kitchen?" Bridget asked as she set the bag on the coffee table before heading to grab some plates.

"Yes, I should be, but I'm taking a break for a moment." Maribelle removed the two sandwich containers from the bag and popped open their lids. "We don't need plates."

"Food always tastes better when it's not eaten in containers." Bridget shoved a plate at her as though she was about to throw it like a discus. "When do you plan to talk to Davis?"

"I don't." Maribelle set the container directly on top of the plate and lifted the B.L.T to her mouth.

"Look, you have to talk to him. I'm sure there was another misunderstanding. The friend comment seems like maybe you overreacted, just as you did with the girl who ran out of gas." Bridget arranged her sandwich on her plate in the shape of a V and dumped the bag of chips neatly in the middle. "He still has your frumpy clothes, and you have his clothes too, so you'll need to see him again anyway."

"I'll swing by his restaurant after the New Year to swap the clothes." Maribelle leaned her head back on the couch pillows. "You know I'd already started to fall for him," She snapped her fingers, "like that. What's wrong with me?"

Bridget placed her hand on Maribelle's knee. "Nothing at all. It's alright to like someone instantly. It's alright to have dates end poorly. But it's not okay for you to spend New Year's Eve with a negative outlook. Besides, I'm not dragging you with me. You should be overjoyed."

"Even if everything was great with Davis, I couldn't make it, too many recipes."

Bridget looked at her cell phone. "It's only six-fifteen. You have twenty-eight hours until the clock strikes us into the New Year."

"I need to sleep tonight and still have eight recipes to go." Maribelle picked up a piece of bacon that'd slid from the sandwich and dropped it into her mouth. "I honestly think if Davis felt any type of connection, he would've reached out to me by now."

"First, he knows you had a lot to accomplish in a short time. Second, we all know guys aren't the best when it comes to follow-through. And third, maybe he thinks *you* don't like him because to me it sounded like you kicked him out before he even finished dinner. And fourth, you ignored him the last time he reached out to you."

"I might have come off a little upset." Maribelle bit her lip. "He said communication was the key to a great first date, so clearly we didn't have it."

"I hate to tell you this—"

"No, you don't." Maribelle shook her head and grinned.

Bridget huffed. "Correct, I don't. You have the habit of jumping to conclusions and misjudging communications. Even you and I had our misunderstandings, for a while until we figured it out and then became best friends."

"You were kind of a pushy girl." Maribelle picked up the other half of her sandwich.

"You always overreacted." Bridget gave her a knowing look, her eyes wide. "I know what your new New Year's goal needs to be." She wiped her lips with a napkin. "To put yourself out there and stop assuming everything with everyone. You told me the recipes are going well and you never expected it because you never tried before. Now it's time, in the New Year, to do the same for yourself."

"What about you, Miss Perfect, what's your New Year resolution going to be?"

"I'm going to take a page from your book, actually. And do something I've always told myself I couldn't do." Bridget smiled wide. "I'm going to learn how to speak French."

"So, you're going to learn French the last week of the next year? That seems like a big task."

Bridget threw her napkin at Maribelle as they laughed. "No, I'm going to start the day after New Years. You've been an inspiration to me. And you know how I keep putting it on the back burner every year."

She knew Bridget was right about putting things on the backburner. Maribelle could be accused of the exact same thing and she needed to put herself out there. Even if not to Davis, but to whomever and overcome her anxiety of assuming she couldn't find love. After all, she did want to get married and start a family before she needed to buy wrinkle cream in bulk. Maribelle would start the New Year fresh, by going to pick up her comfy clothes from Davis and drop his off.

"Does this mean I'm forgiven for missing the New Year's Eve celebration at the beach?"

"As long as you promise to completely and utterly play-up Valentine's Day to an extreme level instead of avoiding it like a witch walking around Salem."

Maribelle groaned. "You know how much I hate Obligatory Flowers and Chocolate Day."

"Well, get your pinks and reds ready, because your Valentine's Day is going to be huge." Bridget danced with her upper body and beamed. "I can see it now, five extreme dates in one day! The set-up of the year."

"No! Absolutely not." Maribelle rolled her eyes. "Trying to kill me with love because you agreed to let me stay home on New Year's Eve and wallow in self-pity is not fair."

"Pilau really was your saving grace, this time. Although, I thought about everything you've been through this year, your dating life, and losing Grams. We could all use a break once in a while." Bridget finished her sandwich and slid her plate onto the coffee table. "But, I do think you should reach out to Davis. Double-check that you didn't take something the wrong way, again." She checked her phone. "I need to get going, picking up a few last-minute items for tomorrow night."

Bridget moved toward the door and pulled on her coat. "Probably best you stay with Pilau anyways. He might react poorly to fireworks." She pulled Maribelle in for a long hug.

"My thoughts, exactly."

Ten

When Maribelle pulled the final dish from the oven, a pecan pie, the clock read eleven forty-five. "Only fifteen more minutes until we say goodbye to this year," she said to Pilau who stood in the kitchen, his nose in the air, taking in the scents. "I can't believe I managed to complete my goal."

Maribelle checked her cell for the millionth time today. Deep inside her heart, she'd hoped Davis would text or call if nothing else to let her know he would be dropping off her clothes. Bridget called about fifteen minutes ago to wish her a Happy New Year's, but she could barely hear her over all the noise around her.

A part of Maribelle now wished she'd gone down to the harbor as she glanced over at the New Year's Eve countdown party on television. She sighed and stared at Pilau.

"Pilau, you want to go to the park? I need some fresh air." Maribelle asked as she headed toward the door. After clipping on the leash, they headed down to the park. Wisps of clouds across a navy black sky provided some shade from the moonlight. A few kids ran past, waving sparklers in the air. She smiled at them, although they didn't see it.

Maribelle found an empty bench and sat down; exhaustion from the week of cooking and baking fell heavy on her shoulders.

"I'm surprised to see you here." A male voice came from nearby. "Shouldn't you be with Bridget at the beach?"

Maribelle's heart fluttered and her fingers and toes tingled at the rush of nervousness. She closed her eyes as if to remember how she looked before she left the house. Her hair was unbrushed, but hopefully resembled beachy waves over a homeless mess. At least Maribelle had brushed her teeth and put on a bra.

Hank came barreling through the grass as Pilau's tail wagged in excitement.

"Shouldn't you be doing something more fun than hanging out in a darkened park?"

"I was hoping to hang out with this woman I met recently. She made me a delicious Chicken n' Dumplings dinner." Davis shoved his hands into his pockets, Hank's leash hung like a scarf around his neck.

"Well, I was hoping to hang out with this chef, but he seemed like he didn't want anything to do with dating anyone." Maribelle fiddled with the cuff of her sweater with one hand and held tight to Pilau's leash with the other.

"That's odd of him because I'm fairly certain he wanted to ask this woman out on a date and possibly kiss her at midnight."

"Wait. What?" Maribelle tilted her head toward Davis. "You mentioned at dinner that you wanted to be friends." She shook her head. "I mean, I don't want to sound full of myself, but I thought we had a nice connection."

"Of course, I want to be friends. That's important in a relationship." Davis reached his hand out and touched Maribelle's elbow, gently holding it.

Maribelle turned toward him and gazed into his eyes. "I'm sorry about the misunderstanding. I keep taking things out of context. Chelsea, and then your friend comment."

Davis placed his thumb on Mariebelle's cheek, brushing a spot of flour from it. "Don't apologize. Let's agree to ask over assume."

A bunch of people nearby shouted happy New Year, as sparklers flittered between the low tree branches. Davis's hand remained on her elbow, as his other hand reached for her waist. Maribelle felt fireworks go off with his touch. She leaned in, and he reciprocated. Pilau, still on the leash yanked her backward. He was playing with Hank behind them, but Davis caught her, both hands on her waist now.

"Happy New Year." The moonlight caught the glimmer in Davis's eyes. "Are you sad we are not at the beach with your friends?"

"Not anymore." She blushed.

"See, it's what friends are for. So how about a date, next week? His face was close enough for Maribelle to breathe in his aftershave.

"I'm definitely free." She smiled. "And I'll cook."

"I can't wait." He leaned in, pausing, their breaths met, matching. When Davis's lips pressed gently against Maribelle's lips, warmth traveled down her neck. She'd been kissed many times, but this kiss was different. There was a want, a need as Davis's lips left hers and then returned before she could get a breath in. Maribelle took a step backward as they separated, dizzy with passion. Davis smiled.

Oh, this New Year is already starting off with a bang.

The Not-Too Shabby Lunch Shake

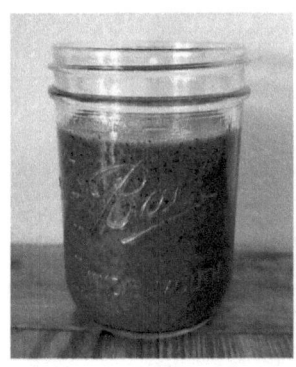

- 1 cup fresh blueberries
- 1 cup spinach
- 1 tablespoon honey
- 4 ice cubes

Blend until smooth

Playlist

Rusted Root – **Send Me On My Way**
Hootie & the Blowfish – **I Go Blind**
Barbie Girl – **Aqua**
Spin Doctors – **Two Princes**
Mariah Carey – **Fantasy**
Backstreet Boys – **Everybody**
Britney Spears – **(You Drive Me) Crazy**
Sophie B. Hawkins – **Damn I Wish I Was Your Lover**
The Proclaimers – **I'm Gonna Be (500 Miles)**

<u>YouTube Link</u>

Acknowledgments

The biggest shout-out to those who made this novella possible.

To you, the reader. Yes, you. Thank you for taking the time to read this book. There are so many authors and books to pick from, and I can't say thank you enough for selecting mine!! **Thank you! Thank you!**

To D.S. and the tireless task of helping make my story as perfect as can be.

To the Kira Stokes Fit App - gosh golly - this app is not only amazingly fun, but it kicked and continues to kick my butt into shape.

To Starla and Rachael - thank you for your support and for being awesome cheerleaders.

And last, but not least, to my dog Ransom, whose endless need for fetch keeps me active a million times a day and also the reason it took so long to write this story.

About the Author

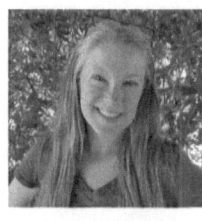 Savannah Hendricks (born in California, raised in Washington, and resides in Arizona) is a full-time social worker and fills as much of her weekends as possible with writing. She loves all things dog-related, has a passion for red wine, gardening, baking, and creating yummy recipes. You'll often find her hollering at the TV during restoration shows when they paint over red bricks.

If you'd love a digital personalized autograph or bookplate, you can request one by visiting: savannahhendricks.com
Please discover more about Savannah by interacting with her on:

Instagram: readingisbetterwithadog
Facebook: AuthorSavannahHendricks

Also By Savannah

Heartfelt Coming of Age/Women's Fiction
My Novel Year
Sun City, 85373 (Multi-Award-Winning)
The Album (Multi-Award-Winning)
I Adopted My Mom at the Bus Station (Multi-Award-Winning)

Humorously Wholesome Romance
Route to Romance
A Hearts of Woolsey series: A Desert Restoration, A Desert Romance, A Desert Rivalry
The Christmas Rental
Grounded in January (Award-Winning)
Grounded in July
To Work Out or to Wed

www.ingramcontent.com/pod-product-compliance
Lightning Source LLC
Chambersburg PA
CBHW030541130626
46552CB00006B/2367